PERFORM & THRIVE

A Sportsperson's Guide to Mental Health and Wellbeing

Sarah Broadhead

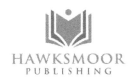

HAWKSMOOR
PUBLISHING

First published in 2022 by Hawksmoor Publishing,
an imprint of Bennion Kearny Limited.

Woodside, Oakamoor, ST10 3AE, UK

www.hawksmoorpublishing.com

ISBN: 978-1-914066-17-7

Sarah Broadhead has asserted her right under the Copyright, Designs and Patents Act, 1988 to be identified as the author of this book. Copyright Sarah Broadhead 2022.

All Rights Reserved. No part of this publication may be reproduced, stored in a retrieval system, or transmitted in any form or by any means, electronic, mechanical, photocopying, recording or otherwise, without the prior permission of the publisher.

Hawksmoor Publishing does not have any control over, or any responsibility for, any author or third-party websites mentioned in or on this publication.

A CIP catalogue record for this book is available from the British Library.

This book is sold subject to the condition that it shall not, by way of trade or otherwise, be lent, re-sold, hired out or otherwise circulated without the publisher's prior consent in any form of binding or cover other than that in which it is published and without a similar condition including this condition being imposed on the subsequent purchaser.

Disclaimer of liability. This book does not contain medical advice. The medical information and any advice or instructions is provided for general information and narrative purposes only. Accordingly, the use, reliance, or implementation of any advice contained within this book is solely at the reader's risk.

Acknowledgements

Many people have supported and contributed to this book, I am grateful they were generous with their time and expertise. I enjoyed interviewing and gaining insights from:

Dame Katherine Grainger, Chris Opie, Annie Last, Matt Walker, Katy Winton, Sheela Hobden, Melissa Luck, Sarah Stevenson MBE, Jade Jones OBE, Hassan Haider, Craig Brown, Rachelle Booth, Charlie Maddock, Gail Emms, Keely Hodgkinson, Marc Woods, Andy Turner, Jordan Thomas, Pippa Woolven, Sarah Hope, Callan O Keeffe, Lauren Williams, Lutalo Muhammad, Craig Morris, Rhys Ingram, Paula Dunn MBE, Wayne Richardson, Jenny Meadows, Trevor Painter, Atholl Duncan, Dr Mike Rotherham, Nick Levett, Gobinder Singh, Dr Duncan French.

Dr Andy Kirkland kindly shared research papers and his wisdom with me.

Dr Peter Olusoga also kindly shared the latest mental health research.

Pippa Woolven provided invaluable feedback on the chapter content as well as encouragement along the way.

Thanks to Rachael Finney for reading chapters and providing articles whilst also studying for her Master's degree in sport and exercise psychology.

Thanks also to my sister Melanie Usman, Lauren Deutsch, and Jayne Ellis for reading and giving feedback.

I wouldn't be working in sport or learnt what I have without the support from Professor Steve Peters and Gary Hall MBE, so many thanks to both.

Steve Ingham, Dan Abrahams, Dr Josephine Perry, and Lyndsey Hall all shared their experience of writing and publishing books which was both invaluable and inspiring. I am grateful to James Lumsden-Cook for providing me with the opportunity to write this book and supporting me at every stage.

Thanks to psychotherapist James Barnes for discussions about mental health and the mind.

I am lucky to have supportive parents, who fostered a love of books and learning from a young age, and family (Mel, Daniel, Erica, and Barnaby). Finally, thank you James for always being there and supporting me in whatever I do.

Sarah

Foreword

My involvement in sport started at the age of eight when my grandad encouraged me to join the local Taekwondo club to keep me out of trouble. Twenty-one years later, I am still competing. The reason I have been able to keep going for so long is because I have learnt how to understand my mind.

Over the years, I have experienced amazing highs and lows from life and sport and realised that it is not enough to work on your body alone. Understanding yourself, and being in the right environment for you, can be the difference between loving your sport or wanting to drop out. I have seen people who got into sport as they enjoyed it, but called it a day as they felt too much expectation and anxiety, or who overtrained and burnt out. With the right knowledge and support, you can avoid these issues.

I first met Sarah when I was 16 years old and joined the Great Britain Taekwondo Academy in Manchester. We worked together for the next ten years, and she has been instrumental in helping me achieve my gold medals at the London and Rio Olympic Games. Sarah helped me become the best version of myself, not just in sport but in life – helping me work out my values and what matters to me. There is no point winning if that is all you have. I was reminded of this after the Tokyo Olympic Games when I initially felt embarrassed that I didn't achieve my goal of a third Olympic gold medal, but – after being inundated with kind messages – I remembered that you are more than your results. There is you, the sportsperson, and you, the person. You need to value both.

This book is important as it will help you to perform at your best without sacrificing your mental health. This is something that I am constantly aware of, and I have learnt how to be open and ask for help from friends, family, and professionals if I am finding things hard. Life does not always go to plan, but there are things you can put in place that can help you cope the best you can. I know how much courage this can take, but avoiding what is going on in our minds doesn't make it go away.

The brain is complex, but this book explains concepts in an accessible, jargon-free way. It will help you understand why you struggle and give you practical methods you can apply straight away. I am pleased that mental health and wellbeing are being prioritised more than ever; by reading this book, you are part of the progress. This book will truly help you to perform and thrive!

Jade Jones OBE
Double Olympic Champion Taekwondo

Table of Contents

Chapter 1: What is Mental Health and Wellbeing? 1

Chapter 2: Culture 17

Chapter 3: Understanding Yourself 35

Chapter 4: Relationships 65

Chapter 5: Managing stress, fear, and anxiety 91

Chapter 6: Physical and Mental Rest and Recovery 125

Chapter 7: Support 147

Appendix: Visualisation 167

Chapter 1: What is Mental Health and Wellbeing?

- What does it mean to be mentally healthy, and how does it link to performance?
- What might you experience if you have poor mental health?
- What causes poor mental health?
- What is the best way to talk about mental health?

There is no agreement on the answers to these questions, so – across this book – I will highlight the differing views of professionals, as understanding these debates will help you decide what resonates best with you... after all, knowledge is power.

Armed with your newfound knowhow, you will feel more confident when talking about mental health, and you will be able to make more informed decisions. My intention is to provide a balanced view and allow you to make up your own mind.

What is mental health?

The term 'mental health' is used a lot more, nowadays, than it was even a few years ago. High-profile athletes such as the gymnast Simone Biles and the swimmer Adam Peaty have done a great job in raising awareness by talking about their experiences.

When you hear the term 'mental health', what does it conjure in your mind? You might think of someone who is struggling or, conversely, someone who is functioning well. It is not always clear what this term means, as it has become a catch-all for many experiences. We are going to explore the differing views of what it means to be mentally healthy and to have poor mental health.

Mental health on a continuum

Continuums or spectrums are one way of looking at mental health, with all of us moving along a sliding scale (sometimes day to day).

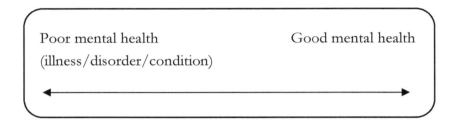

Good mental health

Let's start with the right-hand side: good mental health and wellbeing. The word mental means 'relating to the mind', and our minds are what enable us to think, feel, and experience the world.

As with many matters relating to the mind, there isn't one universally-agreed definition or an objective way of measuring it (that's what I find fascinating about psychology). We must rely on our subjective view of what we are experiencing.

Sometimes health is described as the *absence* of illness/disorder; however, the World Health Organisation says it is more than that. Their definition is "a state of wellbeing in which the individual realises their own abilities, can cope with the normal stresses of life, can work productively and fruitfully, and is able to contribute to their community."[1]

This definition has been criticised for not considering that you can be mentally healthy and experience a range of emotions such as sadness and anger, and not just those associated with wellbeing. It is also full of value judgements, such as the need to work productively to be mentally healthy!

---

[1] https://www.who.int/news-room/fact-sheets/detail/mental-health-strengthening-our-response

Other definitions include emotional, psychological, and social wellbeing, covering things like:

- Satisfaction with life
- Recognising, expressing, and managing your emotions (acknowledging that healthy people may experience human emotions such as fear, anger, sadness, and grief)
- Feeling at peace/content
- Feeling/behaving in line with your own values and beliefs
- Feeling positive and optimistic about life
- Having a harmonious relationship between body and mind
- Using your abilities in line with the values of the society you live in
- Having social skills and functioning in social situations
- Being flexible and coping with adverse life events
- Having a sense of emotional and spiritual wellbeing
- Having meaning in your life

The charity MIND describes good mental health as being generally able to think, feel, and react in ways that you need and want to live your life. This is probably the simplest and most straightforward definition of them all.

All these aspects are subjective; one person's view of coping with adverse life events could be different to someone else's. Looking at that list, it would seem unlikely that any of us can tick *all* those boxes on any given day! Any definition will also inherently contain views of what *society* thinks is good or acceptable.

Being at the far right-hand end of the spectrum – and experiencing emotional, psychological, and social wellbeing – can be described as "flourishing", a term coined by the positive psychologist Martin Seligman.

Another view is that mental health and mental illness are related, but distinct dimensions exist (see the diagram overleaf).

In this, you could have mental illness symptoms/a diagnosis but still have positive mental health and flourish. And vice versa.

This model uses concepts such as diagnosis and illness, which we will explore in more depth later in this chapter.

Two Continua Model [2]

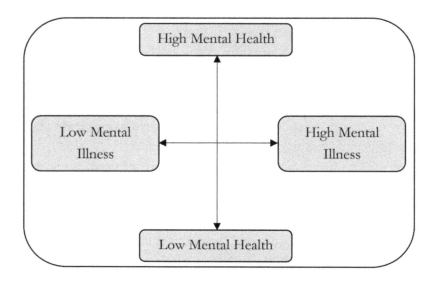

Athlete views about being mentally healthy

For this book, I asked several leading athletes and former athletes what being 'mentally healthy' means for them:

Andy Turner (Track and Field) "Able to enjoy life; can still have worries or doubts though."

Callan O'Keeffe (Motorsport) "Having balance in my life; being self-aware."

Gail Emms (Badminton) "Having balance and perspective."

Katy Winton (Mountain Biking) "Having the capacity to do what I want to do – speak to friends, feel happy, do something nice and not feel bad about it; smile a bit more."

Sarah Stevenson (Taekwondo) "Being able to look forward to things in the future."

Rachelle Booth (Taekwondo) "Able to wake up and want to live a normal life; have goals; feel like I have a purpose, content."

---

[2] Keyes, 2005.

Katherine Grainger (Rowing) "Feeling balanced and able to take things on and cope. Generally upbeat and able to look at the day ahead and look forward to the challenge."

Lutalo Muhammad (Taekwondo) "Clarity. Clear on my goals and where I am going."

Good mental health and wellbeing and performance

Where we are on the continuum influences how we think, feel and act, how we deal with demands, relate to others, and how we make decisions. If you spend periods of time towards the left of the continuum, it can have negative impacts on your ability to train, perform, and recover from illness and injuries.

Whilst you might still be able to perform how you want if you are struggling mentally, being mentally healthy means you are able to *sustain* those performances over longer periods of time, and they are much more enjoyable. Many athletes say they perform at their best when they are towards the right-hand end of the continuum. It allows you to access the automatic physical movements that you have spent hours practising, which is harder to do when you are having mental difficulties. You will be able to get the best out of yourself and enjoy life more if you take steps to work on your mental health. Lutalo Muhammad describes how wellbeing helps him perform at his best. "When I am enjoying life and training, am clear on my goals, and don't want to be anywhere else, the performance benefit is huge. I can't wait to perform."

Activity

So, what is *your* definition of good mental health? It's *your* definition that counts.

What would being mentally healthy, or flourishing, look like for you? How would it help your performance and life satisfaction?

It is helpful to think about this. In doing so, we can get real about mental health. For example, if we feel healthiness is only about experiencing 'positive' thoughts and emotions, then it is *unlikely we will ever achieve this*. In turn, we might think something is 'wrong' with us if we are not happy all the time, and this could be a source of distress.

You can also use your definition of mental health to guide you toward strategies that might help you achieve this. For example, if feeling and behaving in line with your own *values* is part of your definition, then figuring them out could be a great exercise to do.

In simple terms, values are the things that are truly meaningful to you, the things that make everything worthwhile.

There has been lots of research into what can help move us towards flourishing (even if it isn't realistic to be like this all the time), so we will explore these ideas as we move through the book.

Some examples of measures of mental health and wellbeing that have been used with athletes include the World Health Organisation Wellbeing Index [3] and the Flourishing Index [4]. When answering these questions, it is important to consider your current life circumstances and context, as they can influence your answers. The Indexes can be used as gauges – where you can check in every so often – but shouldn't be used as diagnostic tools.

Poor mental health

Poor mental health is an umbrella term that can incorporate other sayings – like mental illness, disorder, or condition – and can describe us when:

- We experience patterns of behaviour, thoughts, feelings, and experiences that result in *significant distress / suffering / pain / damage to health, or which are unusual*
- They impact our life *over a prolonged period*
- Our *normal ways of coping are not working*

However, there is no clear, objective line to cross that enables us to effortlessly identify our experiences of the above.

---

[3] https://www.psykiatri-regionh.dk/who-5/Documents/WHO-5%20questionaire%20-%20English.pdf

[4] https://hfh.fas.harvard.edu

Knowing *when* and *if* something should be described as an illness or disorder is the source of many heated debates. Is the worry you feel a normal reaction to life events… or a disorder? I will show you the different ways we can view these experiences.

Some examples of what other people experience can shine a light on our situations. The International Olympic Committee Mental Health Consensus Statement 2019 reported many of these common experiences amongst elite athletes.

Thoughts and feelings

- High or low moods, or mood swings
- Feeling worthless
- Feeling unable to cope and overwhelmed
- Feeling anxious, fearful
- Panicky
- Not enjoying things that you would normally enjoy
- Loss of hope for the future
- Feeling numb
- Suicidal thoughts and acts

Behaviours

- Avoiding activities or people
- Lack of energy
- Very high energy
- Changes to eating patterns or appetite such as restricting, overeating, binging, and purging (which can sometimes result in dramatic weight change)
- Extremes of behaviour
- Using drugs or alcohol excessively
- Gambling excessively
- Changes to sleep patterns
- Carrying out rituals
- Self-harm

Experiences

- Hearing voices
- Hallucinations

- Having nightmares
- Having flashbacks

If you, or anyone you know, has experienced any of these, you will be aware how confusing, scary, debilitating, and painful they can be. One athlete I spoke to, who was binging and purging food said, "Initially, I didn't think I had a problem. I had to make weight and put myself under pressure to do well, so this helped me to cope and to keep my weight down." This comment is telling since we might not always recognise when there is a problem, especially if it is helping us survive.

What can cause suffering, and what is the best way to view it?

It matters that we understand the different approaches to mental health, so we can decide which ones we relate to. There is no 'one size fits all'; each approach has different ways of making sense of suffering and offers different solutions.

Most people agree that how we experience the world is a complex interaction between what happened to us in the womb, the genes we inherited, our childhood and life experiences, our current circumstances, and the society we live in. What they do not agree on is the best lens to view everything through.

I will discuss two approaches:

The medical model. This uses the same model as physical health, and often gives you a diagnosis.

Non-medical model. This does not believe suffering should be seen as an illness or disorder, but rather as an understandable response to life experiences.

The medical model

This approach describes suffering and distress as an illness, disorder, or condition. It uses the same language and approach used by doctors in other areas of medicine – such as symptoms, patient, and treatment – and is administered in settings such as hospitals and clinics by doctors and psychiatrists.

The medical model believes it can treat emotional suffering and pain, citing perceived advantages, such as people's trust in doctors and their codes of ethical conduct. Medics can see a larger number of people due to the use of diagnosis and psychiatric drugs such that – when services are under pressure – it is argued that this provides the most help to the largest number of people.

Psychiatrists will often carry out history taking and mental state examinations when they meet a patient. This involves gathering information about their life and family and observing them. This information can be used to create a hypothesis about what is wrong, how it got that way, and what can be done about it. They can also use a framework such as the *biopsychosocial approach* to help with this, which is where they consider biological, psychological, and social aspects of a person's life to help make sense of what is going on.

Those using the medical model can provide a diagnosis[5] if they see fit. As part of this process, the medical professional should first rule out purely biological causes (e.g., head injury) or medication side effects. In large parts, the medical community – as with physical health – views diminished mental health as an illness or condition that can be treated. The equivalence between mental and physical health, however, has been challenged more and more in recent years.

Those who oppose the medical model argue that using medical language leads people to believe there is something wrong within their brain/body that needs fixing and, furthermore, that the medical approach has led to widespread overdiagnosis of normal human experiences.

Conversely, many people report that they get benefits from seeing themselves as having an illness and receiving a diagnosis, and want to see their suffering in this way. This is the dominant view in the western world.

Pros of a diagnosis

- It simplifies things by providing a shorthand (as humans, we like to put things into boxes to make them easier to understand)

---

[5] A diagnosis is a way of identifying an illness or disorder from its signs and symptoms.

- It can validate experiences as there is a medical authority attached to it. This can mean others take it more seriously (distress must be real if you have a diagnosis)
- It can help the person make sense of their experiences and give hope that things will improve
- It can help others understand your experiences
- It can feel easier or safer to share a diagnosis than disclose personal experiences
- You might connect with others with the same diagnosis who might share similar experiences
- It is often needed to get access to support such as benefits or therapy, and people may be more likely to get support if they are seen to have a health problem rather than a social problem

Cons of a diagnosis

- They are descriptive rather than attempting to explain causes (and possible causes are not always explored)
- It can place the dysfunction in the individual (for example, someone experiences bullying or abuse at the hands of someone else, causing them emotional suffering. It could be harmful to say they have a disorder when there is an external cause)
- The use of categories is increasingly being criticised, as few people fit neatly into one category
- Several critics have argued that diagnoses medicalise conditions that should only be considered normal life problems
- Often practitioners don't agree on a diagnosis, so you can end up with multiple ones
- Those with the same diagnosis can make sense of their experiences in very different ways
- Some labels can be less socially acceptable than others (for example, schizophrenia)

Non-medical model

This approach is not there to give you a diagnosis. It sees you as a person with a problem rather than a patient with an illness.

Different methodologies can be used, such as formulation (what is wrong, how it got that way, and what can be done about it), psychodynamic (understanding your psychological drives and processes), or narrative-based (creating a story of your life), amongst others. Rather than thinking 'what is wrong with you', the non-medical model focuses on *'What has happened to you?'* [6]

In the narrative approach, for example, you would be encouraged to make sense of *why* you might be suffering distress by creating your story and taking meaning from it. One of the main people behind the narrative approach – Lucy Johnstone – argues that this process is enough; you don't need to label your experiences or see them as an illness. All experiences, behaviours, and thoughts – even extreme or unusual ones – are seen as understandable at some level (even if they don't seem to make sense immediately).

Importantly, this approach doesn't recognise a separate group of people who are mentally ill; it applies to all of us. "Rather than saying we all have mental health, we could say we all have feelings, and at times, those feelings can be overwhelming."[7] In other words, we all experience poor mental health to some degree.

The narrative approach would ask questions such as:

- What has happened to you?
- How did it affect you?
- What sense did you make of it?
- What did you have to do to survive?

This approach is criticised by supporters of the medical model who argue it is impractical to use in the healthcare system.

---

[6] Power, Threat, Meaning Framework. Lucy Johnstone, Mary Boyle, John Cromby, David Harper, Peter Kinderman, David Pilgrim and John Read.

[7] Power, Threat, Meaning Framework. Lucy Johnstone, Mary Boyle, John Cromby, David Harper, Peter Kinderman, David Pilgrim and John Read.

What factors influence our mental health?

It is complicated. We know that there are many factors that can play a part, and they can interact in ways we don't fully understand. Research has found the following factors can play a role:

Social factors

We come into the world with our brains ready to be moulded to our environments. Unlike other animals who are self-sufficient soon after birth, we need to be looked after. That's the price we pay for having brains that can adapt and learn from those around us. This means that *where* we grow up and *how* people care for us – as we develop – have a huge impact on how we function and see the world.

Social factors can influence our personality, brain, and body as we are growing up, and the following highlights some of them that can lead to emotional suffering.

- Adverse childhood experiences (ACEs) such as verbal, physical, or sexual abuse, parental separation, witnessing domestic violence, alcohol and drug abuse, having a parent in prison
- Low socioeconomic status (the education, income, and job role you and your family have)
- Discrimination such as racism and homophobia
- Abuse
- Bullying (including cyberbullying)
- Trauma (for example, a terrifying or distressing event/s)
- Loss of a loved one
- Social isolation and loneliness
- Societal expectations (how you should look, behave, fit in)

It is no surprise that those who live in poverty will struggle mentally as the most basic need – the need to survive – will be under threat. Children and adults living in British households in the lowest 20% income bracket are 2-3 times more likely to have poor mental health than those in the highest.

For athletes, social factors in and out of sport have a huge impact on mental health. Good relationships can help you flourish, whilst poor ones can have the opposite effect. Aspects of sport such as the sporting environment, the expectation to get results, and selection were reported as a source of stress by many of the athletes I spoke with. The mental toll that the Covid pandemic has taken on many of us also highlights the importance of social factors on how we feel.

Chapter 2 will explore, in more detail, how important our environments are for our mental health and how we can optimise the sport setting.

Psychological factors

This covers aspects such as:

- Your personality
- Your emotional development
- Coping strategies you have
- Patterns of thinking, feeling, and behaving
- Your identity and purpose

We all see and interact with the world in our own unique way. Chapter 3 will explore this in more detail, looking at how we can *understand ourselves better* and use this knowledge to help us flourish.

Biological factors

We can't separate our brains from our bodies; therefore, our biology will always be inextricably linked with how we think, feel, and act. There isn't agreement about how much of an impact these factors have – for example, some researchers believe genes play a big role in determining who will suffer, whilst others see it as only being a small part of the picture – but genes need an environment to be able to express themselves, so some argue that the expression of a gene is not inevitable. The brain is the most complicated organ in the body and the most poorly understood.

What is happening in our nervous system and endocrine system (hormones) clearly play a role, and traumatic life experiences have been shown to change the functioning of the brain. We know that lifestyle factors such as sleep, what we eat and drink, and how much recovery we get can also influence our bodies and minds. How these impact on our mental health and ideas for managing them are covered in Chapter 6.

Bringing these factors to life

Louise first picked up a tennis racket at four years old, and she loved it. Her parents couldn't drag her away from the court. Her playing became more and more structured, and she was praised by family and coaches when she won matches. Her family were high achievers, and she said she felt pressure to achieve at something.

From a young age, she liked to do things 'perfectly' and would beat herself up if she didn't. There wasn't much time for socialising with friends as she spent most of her time practising.

At 15 years old, she went abroad to train, only seeing her coach and physical trainer. She felt it was a great opportunity, so she couldn't tell people she was struggling and lonely, and no one asked. When she talked about quitting, everyone said it would be a waste of talent. She often got injured, leading to feeling down and demotivated. She liked the idea of being a top player rather than the reality. She would punish herself by not eating properly or doing extra training when she felt she wasn't doing well enough. She wasn't sleeping very well and rarely took a day off training when not injured for fear of getting left behind in the rankings.

Louise's story highlights how several social, psychological, and biological factors came together to influence how she was feeling. Mapping these out would be the first step in creating a plan to help her become mentally healthy (whatever that means for her).

Summary

- We can see poor mental health and good mental health as being on a spectrum that we move along, or as related but distinct dimensions
- There is no agreement on what it means to be mentally healthy, but most definitions include emotional, psychological, and social wellbeing
- Being mentally healthy means you can experience a range of emotions, not simply being happy all the time
- You can come up with your own definition of good mental health and wellbeing
- Working on your mental health and wellbeing will help your performance and life satisfaction

- We can see poor mental health through a medical or non-medical lens. There are pros and cons of having a psychiatric diagnosis, and it should be an informed choice
- There is no one cause of poor mental health. Factors that play a part include social, psychological, and biological. Taking all these into account to make sense of your experiences can help work out the best solution for you

Chapter 2: Culture

- What impact does the society we live in have on our mental health?
- What is a harmful or healthy culture in sport?
- What can sports environments do to help us thrive?

Sadly, there are many examples of toxic sports cultures that have allowed terrible things to take place. One such culture saw the sexual abuse of young girls in the US gymnastics team, and 500 survivors of abuse came forward during the investigations. Simone Biles said that she not only blames the doctor, Larry Nasser, but the whole system that enabled it to happen.

Pervading culture can have a huge impact on how we function, and the Paralympian Tanni Grey-Thompson wrote a Duty of Care in Sport Review in 2017[8] questioning whether welfare and safety were getting the priority they deserve. As she pointed out, 'Sport has a moral and legal obligation to care for its participants.'

Despite this report, the subsequent Whyte Report, which was released in June 2022, shared distressing experiences from young British gymnasts that included physical and emotional abuse, showing that more work needs to be done to provide healthy environments.

Whilst we bring our own life experiences and personality into an environment, and people can still struggle mentally in the healthiest of environments, it is vital that those in positions of power take their duty of care seriously. It is not reasonable to expect individuals to take sole responsibility for their mental health, and any organisation that professes to care about this – but which doesn't look at its own ways of working – is paying lip service to it. Being part of a healthy sporting environment can be

---

[8] https://www.gov.uk/government/publications/duty-of-care-in-sport-review

positive and life-changing, developing you as a person, so let's look at what can make a culture healthy and unhealthy.

Society

Sport sits within society, and the portrayal of athletes in the media has been shown to play a role in mental health, as well as the general societal expectations we all face.

The first thing to question is whether the modern world has become more difficult, or that we are just getting better at talking about our problems. Every generation will struggle with how society operates to some degree, but it is argued that the world today is more individualistic than ever before, and we have lost a sense of community.

Success is associated with the feeling you must *constantly* achieve more than you did before. If you work hard enough, you can make it, irrespective of luck, privilege, or misfortune.

We have more access to other people's lives through social media, so comparison is common, and we can feel the expectation to live up to certain standards. This can be about how we should look, behave, or what we should achieve by a certain age. Discrimination based on race, gender, faith, disability, sexual orientation, financial status, and more, still exists, of course, and has been shown to cause mental suffering in those subjected to them.

Media and social media

Athletes can sometimes be portrayed as being superhuman by the media, and not allowed to make mistakes or struggle. Being an athlete who 'wins' is highly prized, reinforcing the view that sport is just about medals and outcomes.

Talking about media pressure, the gymnast Simone Biles said, "I truly do feel like I have the weight of the world on my shoulders at times. I know I brush it off and make it seem like pressure doesn't affect me but, damn, sometimes it's hard." In turn, the swimmer Simone Manuel said, "Please stop interviewing an athlete after a disappointing performance. It is mentally and emotionally exhausting to coherently answer questions while trying to process the fact that people already saw you fall short of the goals you worked so hard for, on the world's biggest stage."[9]

Setting commentators abuzz, Naomi Osaka declined the press conferences at the French Open in 2021 as she was worried about the impact it would have on her mental health and was subsequently fined and threatened with exclusion. She withdrew, sparking a debate about the obligations of athletes and the duty of care of organisers.

The more that high-profile athletes talk to the media about themselves as people, the more likely the superhuman myth will shatter. The swimmer Michael Phelps has talked openly about depression and suicidal thoughts, and how he used drinking to cope. His documentary 'The Weight of Gold' explores the challenges that Olympic athletes face. Serena Williams has talked about her experiences of depression and how she works with her support network to help her through those times.

Most people use social media on a regular basis, and for some, it is a necessary part of their sponsorship or team agreement, or a way to gain sponsorship. You might love it or loathe it, but it is unlikely to disappear from our lives. Positive aspects can be connections with like-minded people, stress relief, and motivation; negative aspects can include vulnerability, procrastination, and loss of sleep.

Many athletes have been the victims of online trolls, and GB hockey player Susannah Townsend, for example, has talked about the abuse she would get if she used the hashtag LGBTQ on social media.[10] Depressingly, there were 12,500 racist tweets and posts sent to the England football team players Marcus Rashford, Jadon Sancho, and Bukayo Saka after the team's loss to Italy in the European Championships in 2021. There is clearly work to be done to address these issues in society. At the Olympics, the British Athletes Commission set up a 24-hour hotline for GB athletes who received online abuse.

---

[9] Faustin, M. *et al.* (2022) Effect of media on the mental health of elite athletes. *British Journal of Sports Medicine*, Vol 56 No 3.

[10] https://www.bbc.co.uk/sport/53642350

Managing media

- Ask for support and help if you are getting abuse online. Don't respond; block accounts and report the abuse to the platform and the police if you feel under threat
- Take control of when and how you use social media. Check how you feel after you have been online, and set yourself limits. Tell others around you, as they can help you stick to those limits. Athletes have told me they often keep off social media on the day or week of competition and straight afterwards. You can use scheduling tools to create posts in advance
- Have responses ready post-performance for people who ask how it went. This can help you feel better prepared to deal with questions rather than coming up with them in the heat of the moment
- Be aware of the expectations you might feel from society. Ideas in this book will help you figure out who you are, what is important to you, and help you manage the expectations of others

Sport cultures

Culture can be described as the way we do things 'around here'.

John Amaechi, psychologist and former professional basketball player, says that culture is defined by the worst behaviour tolerated. A team, sport, or club can have great value statements, but if people are allowed to behave in ways that go against these values, they mean nothing. If you go into a club or team, you should be able to describe the culture based on the language you hear, how people speak to each other, what is encouraged and rewarded, and what is punished or ignored.

Activity

Write down three words that describe the culture of the sport, team, or training group you are part of.

Unhealthy cultures

A 'win at all costs' approach is often cited as a driver for unhealthy cultures. If the outcome is so important – and takes on life and death seriousness – toxic behaviours can result. Fear can be at the root of this. This could be a fear of consequences such as the shame of losing, relegation, loss of funding or jobs, and media scrutiny. In some environments, this has resulted in:

- Extreme ways of losing weight or under-fuelling
- Overtraining or training through injury
- Hiding physical or mental struggles (putting on a brave face)
- Fear of failing, feeling relief rather than enjoyment at winning

Non-accidental violence

- Psychological abuse
- Physical abuse (including doping)
- Sexual abuse
- Neglect (failure to meet physical and emotional needs, or failure to protect from harm)

Non-accidental violence happens due to an abuse of actual or perceived differentials in power (IOC consensus statement 2019). Those found to be most at risk are child athletes, athletes who identify as lesbian, gay, bisexual, transgender or queer, and athletes with disabilities.[11]

The reported prevalence of abuse in sport ranges from 2% to 49%, and the impact on individuals can be devastating.[12] Thinking about people that have been subjected to these cultures leaves many people feeling sad and angry; sport should provide positive, not traumatic, experiences!

---

[11] Australian topflight footballer Josh Cavello is the only football player in the world to come out as gay, in 2021.

[12] Reardon, C. *et al*, (2019) Mental health in elite athletes: International Olympic committee consensus statement. *British Journal of Sports Medicine*.

Power

When developing this book, several athletes talked about the difficulties of entering an environment as a young person, and not having the confidence to stand up for themselves or challenge what they were told by someone in power. Older athletes also mentioned power dynamics in their relationships with leaders and coaches.

Power can come from someone's position in a team or organisation, from their knowledge and experience, or from the use of non-violent aggression. They might have power over decisions such as selection, keeping you on funding, access to support, time off, attention and praise, training programmes, etc. A comment from a leader in a position of power can etch itself into the mind of an athlete for a long time. If those in power don't recognise this, it can have a negative impact on those around them. It might not be intentional, but there is a responsibility to be aware. Several athletes have set up 'Global Athlete', which is an international athlete-led movement whose aim is to address the balance of power between athletes and administrators. They are looking to gain more of a voice in world sport matters, and how sport is run.

Examples of unhealthy cultures

Pippa is an endurance athlete who moved to the US to study and train, and she describes the impact the culture had on her: "It was the perfect storm; I had moved away from everyone I loved at home in the UK, was living in a house with people with eating disorders, and in a training group that valued numbers over everything.

"The coach was paid based on our results, and she liked to control everything we did. We couldn't have hobbies or sit in the sun as it would impact on our performance. No one ever asked how you were, and many of the group were extremely thin.

"Those I was living with were getting good times, so I thought how they were eating and living was normal, after a while. You feel abnormal if you don't restrict what you eat.

"If I had a bad race, the coach and others in the group would take it personally. There was nothing we had control over, so monitoring and restricting food was something I could control. If you had a niggle, you were whisked off to the physio bed and given the time off you needed, but no one felt safe enough to tell anyone they were struggling mentally."

Through support and advice from her family, Pippa realised the environment wasn't healthy, and she went back to the UK. Pippa learnt that restricting food, so you don't have the energy needed, is called RED-S (Relative Energy Deficiency in Sport).[13] In the short term, weight loss can lead to performance enhancement, but the long-term health and performance effects can be devastating. We will look at this in more detail in Chapter 6.

Azeem Rafik, who played cricket for Yorkshire CCC, was subjected to racial harassment and bullying whilst at the club. He shared how these experiences impacted on him emotionally when he spoke at a select committee hearing in 2021. He said racist comments were accepted and justified as banter, and no one in power stamped it out. Banter is a common term used in sport, and is often used to justify behaviour; but if the person receiving it sees it as hurtful, then it is not ok.

The anti-bullying alliance[14] describes bullying as being hurtful, repetitive, intentional, and involving an imbalance of power (e.g., someone in a position of power – such as a coach – or a teammate doing it in front of others), whereas banter is a playful and friendly exchange of teasing remarks. If one person is not finding it friendly or playful, then it is not banter. There is no excuse for someone carrying on if you tell them that you see their comments as hurtful.

Duty of care

Duty of care is a moral and legal obligation to ensure the safety and wellbeing of others. Everyone has the right to enjoy sport that is free from harm and abuse, so your club or organisation must satisfy this duty. They need to be able to properly spot concerns and risks and act upon them, and physical and mental health must

---

[13] https://www.red-s.com/

[14] https://anti-bullyingalliance.org.uk

be a priority. There should be a safeguarding policy that is available and understood by everyone.

The Ann Craft Trust[15] has resources available that can help with governance and policies. As an athlete, you should know who you can go to if you are experiencing harm or see it happening to someone else.

Healthy sport cultures

We will look at two areas of a sports culture that can contribute to good mental health and performance. These can apply at youth/development level right through to high-performance sport.

1. Approach to sport
    - Focus on the process
    - Keeping it fun
    - Balance
    - Recognising more than the outcome

2. Understanding and getting the best out of each other
    - Feeling socially connected
    - Shared creation of the culture

Approach to sport

We have seen the potential consequences of a 'win at all costs' culture, so what are the alternatives? Outcomes will always be important in competitive sport, but it is *how you frame them* that matters.

Focus on the process

Cultures can sometimes talk more about the process and 'being the best we can be' rather than the outcome. There will always be consequences to outcomes in life, but focusing on them can promote fear and stress responses, which in turn reduce the chances of performing well over the long term.

---

[15] https://www.anncrafttrust.org/

We cannot directly control an outcome, so focusing on the aspects we *can* control or influence under the circumstances has been shown to help reduce feelings of pressure.

Athletes in cultures that promote this have said, "I felt like I couldn't fail as my coach encouraged me to try to see what happened. We would learn something… no matter what. I don't remember us talking much about medals, just progression."

Others have described how their team took the opposite approach and how unhelpful it was. "I would complete my race, and the team would ask why I hadn't got a better result. I wanted to do well and had given it my all, and – rather than exploring things we could learn or improve for next time – they just talked about the outcome."

Keeping it fun

Sport can be tough at times, but several athletes talked to me about the importance of remembering *why* you got into the sport and the value of having fun. "I have been on a number of professional teams in my career, and I always performed best when the team had a fun vibe. People seemed more relaxed, and you pick up on this."

Often, we get into sport as it is enjoyable, and this can get lost along the way as everything becomes more serious. In fact, it can become a big reason why people drop out of sport. Healthy cultures remind us of what we love about the sport and that we *can* have fun along the way. Shaun White, the Olympic snowboarder, took part in his fifth games in Beijing in 2022. He said that if he didn't *love* what he did, there was no way he would have kept competing for so long.

Team enjoyment has also been shown to enhance resilience, with teams that collectively – not just individually – experience positive feelings proving increasingly motivated to deal with adversity.[16]

---

[16] Sarkar, M. & Page, E. (2022) Developing individual and team resilience in elite sport: research into practice. *Journal of Sport Psychology in Action*.

Balance

The word obsession gets used a lot in sport, and some argue you must be obsessed with what you do to win. There is no denying that a huge amount of hard work and commitment is needed, but if taken to the extreme, it can be counterproductive.

A healthy culture can encourage you to see yourself as more than just an athlete, and a healthy culture actively supports other activities. Fear can be a barrier to encouraging this; a worry that other things will be a distraction to performance. We are not talking wild parties every night here, just doing something that lets you switch off from your sport without feeling guilty, and which allows you to develop other areas of your life and identity.

Some athletes report being happy, with sport being their only focus and they don't feel they are missing out. This might be the case when they are getting the results they want, but when performance dips, or they leave their sport, this approach can be unhelpful.

There are a growing number of athletes that have found improvements to their performance and happiness by having balance in their life. Katherine Grainger, ex-Olympic rower and the Chair of UK Sport, told me how important balance was to her as she completed a PhD alongside her rowing career. "Studying helped me have a different focus and environment, and one benefited the other. I had a coach who encouraged this, and we would talk about what I was working on over coffee. It would have been hard if they weren't supportive of this."

Callan was a junior Red Bull motor racing driver and is now a coach. He recalls how he failed to find balance. "I got myself so stressed; I was too obsessed and didn't need to be. I was weighing out all my food, didn't have a social life, felt guilty if I did anything not related to sport. It was fine when results were going well, but when they weren't, I had nothing else.

"I needed someone to encourage me to find balance as it is hard to do it yourself. I realise now I would have been a better driver if I had found life balance earlier on."

Lizzie Yarnold, ex-Olympic skeleton athlete, took golf lessons and learnt to bake to develop other interests in her life. Sporting careers don't last forever, so developing other skills and interests are vital. Cultures can help people to broaden the number of areas we attach importance to.

Recognising more than the outcome

Cath Bishop,[17] ex-GB Olympic rower says that podium moments don't happen that often, so cultures should emphasise other aspects as being important. These could be learning to deal with setbacks, focusing on improvements, learning about new cultures when you travel, inspiring others, and adding value to your community.

Katherine Grainger says that winning is not a bad thing, and we should be proud to talk of our successes, but it shouldn't be the only thing we talk about. "Athletes should leave their sporting career feeling it was a good use of time and they are better for it... no matter what results they got."

Another athlete told me, "If you didn't get a good result, people would ignore you and gravitate to those who had done well. If you were on a run of poor performances, this could really get you down. Once you started to do well, they wanted to know you again. When you do well, you need less support; it is when you haven't performed how you want to that you need the most help."

A healthy environment will not just celebrate medals, and it won't ignore you if you don't perform to the expected level. Paula Dunn, Head Coach for the British Paralympics programme, described how she created a healthy culture at the Tokyo Paralympic Games. "We had a WhatsApp group. I didn't want to just congratulate those who won medals, so we recognised people who had got season's bests or personal bests, or those who had overcome difficulties to even get to the games."

Sarah Stevenson, GB Taekwondo fighter, told me, "I lost both my parents to cancer in the lead-up to the 2012 Olympic Games. I fought badly but would rather have competed than regret not doing it. It kept me going and gave me a focus. I wouldn't have got to read the Olympic oath or got an MBE if I didn't go. If it was just about medals, I would have felt like it was a waste of time,

---

[17] https://cathbishop.com/the-long-win/

but it gave me so much. You will fail more times than you will win, so you need to learn to manage that."

Understanding and getting the best out of each other

We are all different, so it is not surprising that some cultures suit some people but not others. However, there are things that can be done to get the best out of *everyone* in an environment. Most humans have a need to feel socially connected to others and feel they have a say in how things are done.[18] In terms of creating a culture, most people like to have some input into this. We will look at each of these in turn.

Feeling socially connected

A positive social connection with a person or group means that you trust them and feel safe enough to be yourself. You don't fear being rejected or shamed if you share your opinions, make a mistake, or take a risk. The psychologist Amy Edmondson calls this 'psychological safety'.

Psychological safety in sport has been defined as 'The perception that you are protected from, or unlikely to be at risk of, psychological harm in sport.'[19] Katherine Grainger endorses this approach. "You should feel safe to be yourself and feel understood as a human being."

In a safe culture, there is no blame. Instead, open discussions are held about what could be improved. This doesn't mean everyone is always happy or avoids tough conversations; in fact, the opposite is true. If people feel safe, it means difficult topics can be talked about without fear of the consequences, and egos are put to one side to do what is best for the common goal. If an athlete feels their selection is under threat if they speak up, then it is less likely they will.

---

[18] https://selfdeterminationtheory.org/theory/

[19] Vella, S.A. *et al*, (2022) Psychological safety in sport: a systematic review and concept analysis. *International Journal of Sport and Exercise Psychology*.

Those in positions of power have the most influence in creating a feeling of safety; they need to be accessible, approachable, and care (people can tell). Being aware of this influence and checking how safe people feel is essential. Encouraging others to speak first before giving their opinion, asking for views different to their own, and praising people when they speak up, all help to create this feeling. When people always agree with those at the top, it is not a good sign.

Katy Winton races bikes downhill. Imagine a slope covered in rocks so steep you can barely walk down it… that is what Katy rides down at speed. "We are doing a dangerous thing, so you need to be in an environment where you feel safe, and people are calm.

"If people around you are stressed, critical, or don't believe in you, you will ride stiff, and results go out the window. Respect and kindness make all the difference."

Psychologically-safe environments ensure positive and respectful relationships between teammates as well. The power isn't always with the top person or captain.

Being in a psychologically-safe sporting environment doesn't mean all obstacles are removed or there are no real-world consequences based on performance. Cultures should help equip people to deal with these and provide opportunities to face tough things in a helpful way. It is not enough to promote health by avoiding stress or building bridges to keep people from falling into the river. Instead, people must learn to swim.[20] In environments where high levels of challenge exist, such as sport, there should be equally high levels of support. Duncan French, Vice President of Performance at UFC, said, "You can't change the bar of what you need to do to perform, but you can help fighters develop skills to navigate it."

Understanding each person as an individual is the key to connection. What drives them, what are their fears, what is important to them in life, what challenges have they faced, what is the best way to communicate with them? A healthy culture can understand, appreciate, and interact with people from cultures or

---

[20] *Unravelling the mystery of health: How people manage stress and stay well.* Aaron Antonovsky (1987)

belief systems that are different to their own. Callan describes how he does this with the drivers he coaches. "As a team, we take an interest in each person's personal life. We make time to go for a coffee outside of training and consciously don't talk about racing."

When everything is measured to the nth degree, it can be easy to forget there is a person behind the numbers. Many athletes talked about wanting to be seen and cared about as a person rather than a cog in a machine. Craig Morris, technical coach for GB Canoe Slalom, believes in a person-centred approach, prioritising connections with the athlete. His approach is praised by athletes he works with, such as Kimberley Woods, who has talked openly about her emotional struggles and self-harm. Morris helped her to feel comfortable enough to be open and helped her find the right support.

Craig Brown, psychologist, and ex-Taekwondo athlete, said that we are missing an opportunity if we don't take time to learn about each other. "I am Christian, and other athletes on the team were Muslims. Having people in the environment that take time to understand what your faith and culture means to you is so important. Representation matters as others of the same race or faith can relate to you more easily."

Hassan Haider, another ex-Taekwondo fighter, agreed, saying, "The Asian culture puts pressure on you to go to University. What I was doing was different, so I felt I had to be successful. Having people in my sport understand this pressure was really helpful."

The concept of privilege has been talked about a lot more in recent years, and how it is important to recognise where we might have it and others don't. John Amaechi summarises this concept brilliantly in his BBC bitesize video[21] where he talks about privilege as being the absence of inconvenience and challenge in a particular area of your life (for example, being wealthy or able-bodied or white). It doesn't mean you have not had challenges or life has been easy, but that your finances, skin colour, or ability were not the cause of your hardship. Healthy cultures will make the effort to understand, avoid defensiveness, and make changes to address inequalities. These should be captured in policies and brought to

---

[21] https://www.bbc.co.uk/bitesize/articles/zrvkbqt

life by actions. Paula Dunn said that, as a team, they remind themselves of the mental toll that travel and accessibility can have for Paralympic athletes, and how they make efforts to understand and support people as well as they can.

Understanding how a female athlete is different, and applying this knowledge in practice, is starting to happen in high-performance sport. Most coaches are male, so they are not aware of – or don't feel comfortable – talking about periods and the impact on training, mood, and performance. Cultures need to support people to feel comfortable having these discussions.

It takes time and effort to understand people and develop relationships, but it is worth it. As Katherine Grainger says, "It brings out the best in people and makes it more sustainable. It is not a healthy culture *or* medals."

Shared creation of the culture

It takes effort, conscious thought, and action to create a healthy team culture. Involving others in the creation usually results in better engagement than just telling people what it will be. For individuals, this could be creating a culture with your coach, family, or supporters. These areas need to be discussed and worked on regularly; this is not a one-off activity! Ideally, you would have a person who can drive this and keep a watch on whether the culture is being lived. Just because everyone comes up with it doesn't mean they don't need reminding or encouragement. When things are not going well, it is particularly important to review progress and make sense of what has happened.

Aspects to discuss when creating a culture:
- What is important to us and why?
- How can we get the best out of each other?
- Approach to sport – what are our views on having a process focus, keeping it fun, balance, and recognising more than the outcome?
- Roles – who will do what?

- Behaviours on and off the field of play – what are acceptable and unacceptable behaviours? How will we deal with conflicts?
- Accountability – how will we remind each other of these factors and hold each other to account in a helpful way?

Aim to be as specific as possible, so rather than saying honesty is important to us, say *how* you will be honest with each other and *when*.

Chris Opie, ex-professional road cyclist, described how a team he rode for would make time to develop their team culture, "At the start of the season, we had a workshop where staff and riders came up with what was important to us and ways of working as a team. We would revisit it throughout the year, and it meant we stayed on the same page. At first, we thought we should just be getting on with riding our bikes rather than sitting in a room, but it helped us feel trusted and valued."

Encouraging conversations about mental health

Creating a psychologically-safe culture is a good place to start if you want people to be open with each other about their difficulties. If people in positions of power (such as coaches) are willing to role model this openness, others are more likely to follow suit. In 2019, 75% of deaths recorded as suicides were male, and suicide rates were higher among young black men than white men. Some argue that the masculine ideal held up by society *and sport* contributes to this, and makes it harder for men to share how they are feeling. Having males in sport who talk about their challenges is vital.

Numerous athletes have highlighted the power of having mentors from their own and other sports. They could be current or retired athletes who can share their experiences plus the lessons they have learnt. Healthy cultures should role model and encourage actions that help promote positive mental health, such as switching off, taking time out, and managing stress (see Chapters 5 and 6).

They should also communicate what to expect if you disclose your struggles. For example, who will be told? What support is available? How will it impact on selection? Knowing this in advance is likely to increase open conversations.

Education about mental health and the continuum discussed in Chapter 1 can help normalise experiences. Providers such as Mental Health First Aid offer training based on the medical model and diagnosis, whereas the organisation Changing Minds have delivered non-diagnostic-based training to Olympic sports.

Mental health screening is used by some high-performance sports alongside physical health checks – often following an injury, before and after major competitions, or before transitions out of sport. The IOC Mental Health Working Group has developed a tool called SMHRT-1[22] that can be used by athletes, coaches, and family members to check how someone is doing mentally. As with any way of measuring how someone is feeling, the person answering must feel safe enough to be open. This should not be used for diagnostic purposes.

The IOC Mental Health in Elite Athletes Toolkit[23] provides a guide to creating a mental health action plan that can demonstrate an organisation or club is taking mental health seriously. The guide can also apply to non-elite clubs.

Summary

- Society and sports cultures can both have an impact on our mental health. Being aware of their influence can help athletes manage it more effectively and pick the environment that suits them best
- Unhealthy cultures can result in non-accidental violence and other damaging practices, often driven by a 'win at all costs' approach
- Healthy sports cultures encourage approaches such as keeping it fun, focusing on the process, balance, and recognising more than just the outcome

---

[22] https://olympics.com/athlete365/app/uploads/2021/06/BJSM-SMHRT-1-Athlete365-2020-102411.pdf

[23] https://olympics.com/ioc/news/ioc-launches-safe-sport-action-plan-and-mental-health-toolkit-for-elite-athletes

- Healthy sports cultures create environments where people feel safe to be themselves and give their opinions. They take time to understand people and address inequalities. When there is high challenge, they provide high levels of support. It is not a case of having a healthy culture or good performance – you can have both! Involving everyone in the creation of a culture will help with engagement
- Finding a mentor from your own or another sport can help you thrive in your environment
- Everyone has a right to enjoy sport free from harm and abuse. You should know who to go to if you experience this or see it happening (ask who the safeguarding lead is)

Chapter 3: Understanding Yourself

- Why is it important to understand yourself?
- How can you understand yourself better and work out what is important to you?
- How does your brain work?

Why is it important to understand yourself?

Humans are complicated. To be human is to have dreams, fears, existential dilemmas, joy, pain, suffering, and conflicting thoughts in your own mind. Despite this complexity, we can still learn about ourselves and gain insights into what makes us tick. It is worth the effort this takes as it can bring benefits such as:

- Working out what matters to you and how you want to spend your time on this planet (so you can make decisions and act in ways that are in line with this)
- Understanding patterns of how you think, behave, and feel (awareness is the first step in being able to change or manage them)
- Understanding your needs and what will help you be mentally healthy
- Finding the right environment and culture for you
- Having more fulfilling relationships
- Being confident in who you are

Several athletes I spoke with stressed the importance of 'knowing yourself' for good mental health and performance. Katherine Grainger, for example, explained how getting to know herself helps her to spot warning signs that things in life have gotten out of balance, which impacts on her mental health.

In turn, Gail Emms, ex-GB badminton player, stated how personal development whilst you are an athlete is helpful later in life, "You are more than just a sportsperson, so get to know you, your personality, behaviours, values. Life will throw stuff at you, but if you know who you are – and how to get the best out of yourself – you can deal with it better."

Sarah Hope, a British wheelchair basketball player, described how learning to understand herself was one of the most helpful things she has done in her life and sporting career. "I knew I was different to the other kids at school, but didn't know why. I remember, aged eight in art class, everyone was saying how all our drawings were good when it was obvious Claire's was the best. I didn't get why they were lying to each other. Over the years, I read more and realised I am autistic, eventually getting a diagnosis aged 30. It has helped me to understand why I find some things hard and how I can adjust for them (for example, wearing noise-cancelling headphones in the supermarket). I can help others understand how I function best, and it helps me avoid the burnout I experienced before I knew how to manage things."

How do you want to be?

Have you ever stopped to think how you would like to be and what is important to you? We will explore this question and look at how our minds can make this more difficult at times.

How you want to be

Values (what is important to you)

The meaning you give your life

Your identity

Your personality characteristics – thoughts, feelings, behaviours

What can help you be like this

Understanding how your brain works

Exploring current patterns and developing self-awareness

Self-awareness and reflection are essential skills to help you be how you want to be and improve your mental health. There are aspects of our minds that we are not aware of, or avoid, and patterns that are automatic, so we don't even realise we are doing them. Only through reflection can we start to understand ourselves. This could be as simple as writing down your thoughts and feelings for a few minutes a couple of times a week.

What is important to you in life?

Being how you want to be is living a life based on what matters to you. What is important to you at the age of 14 might be very different to when you are 40, so this is a lifelong question to consider.

What is important is often called your values. Taking time to work out what is important to *you*, how you want to spend your time and money, and what your view of life success is can be helpful if you want to improve wellbeing and make better decisions. A palliative nurse recently collated the top five regrets of the dying, which were: [24]

1. I wish I'd had the courage to live a life true to myself, not the life others expected of me
2. I wish I hadn't worked so hard
3. I wish I'd had the courage to express my feelings
4. I wish I had stayed in touch with my friends
5. I wish that I had let myself be happier

Spending time considering your values and behaving in line with them reduces the chances of having regrets later in life.

Whilst deciding on your values, you should do the following:

- Think about times you have been proud of yourself or felt most fulfilled
- Think about people you admire and respect. What do you value in them?
- Think about your moral code. Do you want to include this (for example, honesty)?
- If you behaved in line with these values, would you feel successful in life?

---

[24] *The top five regrets of the dying: a life transformed by the dearly departing.* Bronnie Ware (2019)

Some things we value can be out of our control – such as achievement or wealth – whilst we have more control over others, such as empathy (we can choose to treat others with empathy). If you choose a value that is out of your direct control, it can be helpful to focus on the process that will help you move in that direction.

Pippa, who we met in chapter 2, said, "I feel as though a lot of athletes are conditioned to feel most proud of their sporting achievements (race wins, PBs) when really, they've come at the cost of other things, like relationships or behaving in a way we aren't proud of (e.g., setting a poor example to others by being so unhealthy).

"For me, at least, other things have brought more pride than my sporting achievements, but I rarely stopped to think about that at the time. It is so important to stop and think about them to figure out what truly matters."

Examples of values

> *Activity*
>
> Highlight the pursuits, overleaf, that you feel are most important to you. You might want to come up with your own that are more relevant to you.
>
> Narrow the list down to 5 or 6 and put them in **priority order.**

Achievement	Kindness
Autonomy	Learning
Balance	Loyalty
Belonging	Mastery
Challenge	Order
Competence	Passion
Competition	Peace
Connection	Persistence
Empathy	Positivity
Fairness	Power
Freedom	Quality
Fun	Relationships
Health	Respect
Independence	Safety
Innovation	Sustainability
Integrity	Variety
Intimacy	Wealth

Sometimes you think you value something highly, but realise later that it's not the most important thing in life, often learning this the hard way. Having a health scare can make you look after yourself. A family member becoming ill can remind you of the importance of spending time with them. If you operate for periods of time in ways that don't fit with what is important to you, life can be draining or unsatisfying. There can be times when one area of your life takes up most of your time and focus – such as exams or a major project – but you can still find pockets of time for your values!

We are social beings who want connections with others and – naturally – what you value can be influenced by what other people think. This can happen before you are even aware… as you are growing up. Developing your own view of the world and deciding what you believe in is part of gaining independence, but it isn't always easy. Being aware of these influences puts you in a better position to decide what matters to you.

Evie Richards is a cross-country mountain biker and has spoken about how she values social relationships. "I thought I couldn't have a social life if I wanted to ride. Now I see you can do both; you can have a life outside of cycling, you can have friends off the bike, but then you can still race well. I was always so worried that if I saw my friends, it would make me slower, but now it makes me faster. You can still have a social life and race fast."[25]

Jade Jones, meanwhile, explained how family is top of her priority list. "I would do anything for my family; I am so protective of them. If I couldn't go home to Wales regularly to see them, I would really struggle."

Activity
1. Write down the times you spend doing things that are in line with your values
2. What do you do that is *not* in line with your values or doesn't follow your priority order?
3. What small step could you take to move yourself closer in line with your values and priority order?

Every so often, revisit your values list and see how you are getting on.

Meaning

Having meaning in your life has been linked to improved mental health and wellbeing, and its absence to feelings of emptiness, hopelessness, and despair.

Working out the meaning you want your life to have is part of the process of understanding yourself. Meaning is defined as *connecting*

---

[25] https://www.pinkbike.com/news/interview-evie-richards-reflects-on-her-rise-to-the-top-in-2021.html

and contributing to something beyond yourself. Four pillars of meaning have been identified as being important.[26]

Belonging – having relationships where you treat each other like you matter and are wanted, and are fully present with each other. Finding a sporting environment where you feel you belong can be an important part of this pillar. Relationships are critical to our mental health, which is why Chapter 4 is devoted to them.

Purpose – this is what gets you out of bed and gives you a focus. This could be a grand purpose like finding a cure for cancer, having a goal, or being a good friend. You must care about it; it must matter to you.

This is sometimes called 'finding your why', and it makes it easier to do tough things if you have a purpose driving you.

A purpose that contributes to something outside of you has been shown to be powerful for improving wellbeing. In a sporting context, this could be overcoming challenges to inspire young people or helping at your local club to develop others. Jordan Thomas, a Karate turned Taekwondo fighter, said helping others find peace and happiness is his passion and helps him mentally. "I volunteer with kids who have been kicked out of school and help out at my club as a karate instructor," he explained.

Outside of sport, this could include doing small things to help others or your community. A great example of an athlete making a difference to others is Marcus Rashford and his campaign for free school meals.

Storytelling – this is how we make sense of our experiences and place in the world. It is all about understanding how *you became you* with the ability to be the author – editing and retelling your story in a helpful way. We can find meaning from difficult times and create the narrative we want. No one would choose hard times over positive life experiences, but people are often surprised by the growth that happens afterwards. From adversity can spring greater appreciation of life, the identification of new possibilities

---

[26] *The power of meaning: the true route to happiness.* Emily Esfahani Smith (2017)

or purpose, strengthened relationships, and enhanced spiritual development.

Sometimes, it can be painful reflecting on your story, and therapy offers a place where you can talk about it, discuss events, and find meaning. You can also do this yourself or with someone you trust.

Callan described the story he told himself and how he was able to change it. "As a junior, I used to win everything; it came easy. As I moved up to senior races, I won a lot less and struggled to deal with the losses. I saw losing as failing, and this really got me down. After I retired and became a coach, I was able to take some meaning from my experiences. It taught me how to handle tough times and learn from them. I now help develop these skills in the drivers I coach."

Transcendence – this is an experience that is beyond the ordinary and forces you to shift how you see yourself and the world. The feeling you get on a mountain top when you feel part of nature and a tiny part of the world is an example of this. Your sense of self diminishes. Becoming a parent can give people this experience and shift their worldview. Andy Turner, former GB track and field athlete, became a father at 23 years old. "This became my reason for being and racing. If I win this race, I can buy a pushchair. I didn't see this as pressure; I turned it into a positive drive."

Coach Pete Carroll from the Seattle Seahawks NFL team says that without purpose and meaning there won't be winning. If you don't have a purpose, you don't know where to put your strengths. His team's purpose is to strive to be the best they can be, as focusing on anything else will frustrate them and they can't control it.

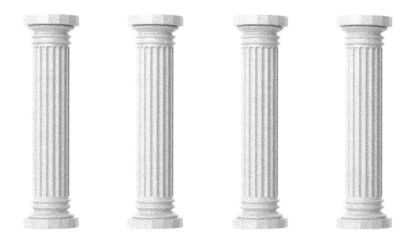

	Belonging	**Purpose**	**Storytelling**	**Transcendence**
Possible actions	Practise being fully present with the person you are with	Do one thing today that helps someone else Write down what is getting you out of bed and excited	Think about the past month. What stories have you told yourself about what has happened and what it means? Is this story helpful?	Go outside into nature and take in your surroundings

Activity

Think about what each of the four pillars means to you. Are there any that you need to pay more attention to and develop?

Identity

Identity is the values, beliefs, characteristics, appearance, and goals that characterise a person or group.

Having an identity can give you a sense of belonging, which we have seen is important for wellbeing. When you meet someone new, what are the first things you tell them about yourself? This can give you a clue about the identity you see as most important.

Identity development often happens during our teenage years when we are working out who we are. This can be influenced by role models, society, and the identity options we see around us. Identity is formed by exploring options and then making a commitment. If we feel confused, we don't have a clear sense of who we are or our role in society.

Identity foreclosure is when we commit to an identity without much exploration or accept an identity chosen for us by others, such as parents, coaches, or teachers. Focusing all our energy on one identity, such as 'being an athlete', can be helpful for committing to training but can have unhelpful consequences, such as overtraining or training through injury. If our whole identity is wrapped up in one area, and this doesn't go well, it can be devastating. It can stop us having balance and mean we feel worthless if we don't do well in our sport or get injured.

Developing *self-worth* can provide a solid foundation for dealing with life's ups and downs and being confident in your identity. Self-worth is the sense that you are good enough and worthy of love from others that isn't dependent on being a certain way or achieving something. If your self-worth is contingent on winning or fitting in, then you might feel worthless if you don't.

If you think about a newborn baby, most of us would say they are valued and have worth. Along the way, we then put conditions on ourselves we must meet to have worth. Developing this unconditional self-worth can be hard if those around you link achievements to being worthy. If you don't have self-worth, it doesn't matter if you are sitting on a yacht in the Mediterranean or winning medals; it won't make up for it.

Tom Bosworth is a GB race walker who was bullied at school for being skinny and gay. He became focused on winning, which had an impact on his relationships with his family and fiancé. He said he didn't know who he was if he wasn't winning. His self-worth was completely tied to how well he was doing, which inevitably was up and down.

In 2018, Tom attempted to take his own life, which resulted in him receiving therapy and – as part of this process – he has re-evaluated where he gets his self-worth from. Tom realised that he is more than just results. He was able to invest time in his relationships again and got a dog to help give balance to his life.[27]

In comparison, Jade Jones, GB Taekwondo fighter, told me, "To be honest, my self-worth has been based on winning at times in my career. I was shy when I was young, and medals made me confident. When I was winning, I felt like a champ; and when I lost, I felt down and insecure. Since losing in Tokyo, it has reminded me to look at it another way. You are more than just an athlete, and young kids need to be taught this. There is you – the athlete – and you – the person – and you need to value both.

"Initially, I felt embarrassed that I had let people down, but everyone was so kind to me and sent lovely messages. I realised people can value you for how you deal with tough times as much as they do for winning. Fighting again and carrying on to Paris for my fourth games shows that I don't give up. Not just getting self-worth from medals means I can enjoy it more and see it as a challenge, which means I fight better."

Keely Hodgkinson, GB 800m runner, says her self-worth doesn't just come from results. "I obviously like the feeling of being the best, but it is also about the journey to getting medals. You are not worthless without them."

> ### *Activity*
> What is your self-worth based on? Is this helpful? Could you adapt it to help improve your wellbeing? Chapter 5 explores self-compassion, which is one way to improve self-worth.

---

[27] https://www.youtube.com/watch?v=PxnCqvQ-Dts

What is your identity? What roles do you identify with? Is one identity or role more prominent than others? What would be the benefits of developing other roles?

You could think of identities such as cultural, spiritual, gender, physical characteristics, sexual orientation, and roles such as friend, son or daughter, sibling, partner, coach, training partner.

How does your brain work?

The brain is the physical matter inside your skull, whilst the mind (which you cannot physically touch or see) is your ability to think and feel.

The neuroplasticity of the brain (its ability to reorganise and respond to life events) is what allows us to make changes and learn new things until the day we die. Every person's brain is unique as no one has had the same experiences as you, so it is not surprising it is the most complex organ in the body.

Let's have a look at how the brain makes sense of the world and *influences* how we think, feel and behave.

Your brain is enclosed in a dark, silent box – your skull – and must try to make sense of what is going on to keep you alive and well. If you get to the end of the day, and you are still alive, it has done its job, even if you have had experiences such as fear or worry along the way.

The brain must work with sensations coming in (sight, smell, sound, etc.) and internal bodily sensations. It makes predictions about what is happening based on past experiences, beliefs, and knowledge and might modify things further, later on, if there is more information (this is how learning takes place). It looks for patterns to work out if you have seen this or something like it before. This happens automatically without us being aware. Most of our lives are spent on automatic pilot. If the brain perceives a threat, a 'fight, flight, or freeze' response will kick in.

The brain is always regulating your body, and your body is always sending sense data to your brain to ensure you don't run out of energy and fail to get what you need. The brain's modelling of the state of your body is experienced as feeling pleasant, unpleasant, calm, worked up, energetic or fatigued. We are not always great at interpreting these signals accurately.[28]

The story of Sam illustrates this.

Whilst growing up, Sam learnt that achievement matters, and that her family interpreted losses as failures to be ashamed of. At competitions, this belief about loss meant Sam saw the situation as threatening. Her brain's prediction, based on past experiences, was that she would not enjoy the competition and would feel overwhelmed. She wasn't aware this was why she felt overwhelmed.

Adrenaline was released in Sam's body, giving a high heart rate, sickness, and sweaty palms, which she interpreted as proof of anxiety and a prelude to something bad happening. Sam found it hard to follow the game plan as she was so focused on the outcome and what would happen if she lost.

When Sam didn't perform as well as she did in training, the reactions of those around her reinforced the belief that this situation felt scary. Sam was chatty outside of competitions but became quiet and withdrawn on the day of the event. Events, themselves, were not objectively threatening, but past experiences and beliefs meant this was how they were perceived. Sam's view of internal bodily sensations backed this up.

It can seem like we have no choice in how we think and feel, at times, but being aware of how we make sense of the world allows us to check if our perceptions are accurate. So, what could Sam do with this knowledge?

High heart rate and sweaty palms are experiences we can have if we are excited. Athletes, such as Sam, can learn to see these as signs they are *ready to perform* rather than nerves. Sam can also learn how to manage these internal sensations through breathing techniques. She could examine beliefs about loss and develop healthier approaches, such as seeing it as an opportunity to learn from mistakes. She could seek out people who will support her in developing helpful approaches and beliefs – focusing on aspects she can control and seeing competitions as a challenge.

---

[28] *Seven and a half lessons about the brain.* Lisa Feldman Barrett (2020)

Sam could also work out her values, self-worth, and the meaning she gives to sport – discussed earlier in the chapter – to develop a stable foundation.

Changing our perceptions is not always an easy process, especially if we learnt to see the world a certain way from a young age. Building awareness of how we see the world is the first step. We don't see things as they are; *we see them as we are*.

Sometimes, the sense we have made of something is right, and we don't need to change our perceptions. But, as much of this happens without us being aware of it, examining and reflecting on the sense you make of the world is helpful. You can do this by regularly reflecting on how you think, feel, and behave in different situations.

Activity

Write down how you see situations such as competitions. What beliefs do you have? Are they accurate and helpful? If not, what can you replace them with? You will need to remind yourself of the new beliefs you want to develop on a regular basis.

Emotions

We know that your brain's job is to keep you alive, and it makes predictions based on past experiences. The emotions you experience are influenced by these predictions. Sam's view of the world contributed to her feeling anxious and overwhelmed. Being able to recognise your emotions and the beliefs that underpin them is a key part of understanding yourself and being how you want to be.

Emotions can get a bad press compared to rational thinking, and we can be taught to hide or control them… but we need to learn to embrace them! There are no good or bad emotions; they are all an amazing insight into what matters to you and how you see the world. If we ignore them and suppress them, they don't go away and can show themselves in ways that are not helpful. It is argued that ignoring emotions can suppress the immune system, for example.

Feeling angry can show that an injustice has happened and fuel a desire to make things better. Anger can sometimes be easier to show than the fear or emotional pain we are actually experiencing, so we need to explore what lies beneath. Showing your emotions to others can help develop meaningful connections.

A good way to develop an understanding of yourself and your emotions is to build your emotional word vocabulary (called emotional granularity). Rather than saying I feel depressed or in a bad mood, develop more specific words that capture how you feel, such as dejected or hurt.

The feelings wheel[29] is great for specific emotion words. Look it up. Once you have described more accurately how you feel, it can be easier to work out why. Develop curiosity about why you have these feelings. Is there anything you can do to change how you feel, or is it appropriate in that situation and you need time to sit with them or talk to someone about how you feel. Do you need to act based on how you feel? Is your perception accurate? Giving yourself time to reflect on your feelings can help you act in ways that you want; ways that you won't regret later.

> *Activity*
>
> Write down the emotions you experience over the course of a day and see how *specific* you can be with the words you use. What can you learn about yourself from these emotions? If the words relate to fear, worry, or being overwhelmed, then Chapter 5 is the place to head.

Rationality

We like to think of ourselves as rational beings, but the reality is this doesn't come easy to us. It is a skill we can develop that will help us to achieve goals, solve problems, and gain perspective.

The human brain has biases that make rationality harder, so we need to recognise them to avoid them. Examples include confirmation bias, where we favour information that matches

---

[29] https://blog.calm.com/blog/the-feelings-wheel

what we already think; or loss aversion, where we register losing something more strongly than gaining it.

To understand yourself, you can examine the biases you have. To improve rationality, we can acknowledge uncertainty, question rather than accept information and thoughts, and change our minds if the facts change. It is a tool that can be used to manage stress and will be discussed in Chapter 5.

Models of how the brain works

Below are two popular models that can help you to understand your brain and summarise what we have just covered. Many athletes say they find benefits in using a model as it simplifies how they understand themselves and provides a language they can share with others.

In his book 'Thinking Fast and Slow', Daniel Kahneman splits the brain into two modes. System 1 is fast and automatic, whilst System 2 is slow, analytical, and logical.

If you have practised something and you can do it without much thought, it is likely to be System 1 in action. If you are learning something new, that would be System 2. If you overthink a skill that is automatic, it can mess it up, so trying too hard is sometimes counterproductive. Trusting the skills and decision-making needed for your sport and letting System 1 run is crucial for performance. You can do this by managing the perception of threat that often prevents System 1 from running (see Chapter 5).

Professor Steve Peters created the Chimp model, described in his book 'The Chimp Paradox.' This model splits the brain into three systems.

1. The Chimp – this part helps you survive, using drives (such as food or sex), emotions, and emotional thinking to help achieve this. It looks out for threats, which can result in fear and anxiety
2. The Computer – this is your automatic beliefs and behaviours based on past experiences. It is the fastest part and is like Kahneman's system 1
3. The Human – this part uses rational thinking and perspective and represents how you want to be

This model reinforces the importance of beliefs and past experiences on how we think, feel, and behave. By changing your beliefs, you can influence your chimp and manage your emotions.

This model encourages you to develop awareness of how each system works for you; for example, working out what your chimp sees as a threat. For Sam, her human wanted to have perspective and enjoy sport. By examining her beliefs and replacing them with new ones, she can help her chimp to see competitions as less scary and more enjoyable. Some athletes find seeing themselves as separate from their chimp makes it easier to manage their thoughts and feelings.

Neurodiversity

This describes the fact that all brains are different. Terms such as autism, ADHD, and dyslexia are used to describe patterns of processing information and interacting with the world. Many people find these terms helpful as it assists them to understand themselves, feel part of a community, and access helpful information.

Sarah Hope, GB wheelchair basketball athlete, describes her experience of autism. "I have sensory sensitivity, so a strobe light feels like being punched in the face and being in a supermarket takes a lot of my capacity to manage. I struggle to process the spoken word compared to something in writing and can end up agreeing to something I didn't mean to on the phone.

"I don't see my brain as being better or worse than others; it is just different. I can communicate with other autistics easily. I have learnt to say what I think I am supposed to say, but I am not always able to recognise what I or other people are feeling. My day-to-day struggles are really just trying to keep up with neurotypical expectations.

"I have a fixed routine, so a sudden change of plans is overwhelming. I can change but not immediately. It is easier to ask for adaptations to be made around my wheelchair, such as putting a ramp out, but people don't always get why you need advance notice of plans or plain language. I take things literally, so I hate the phrase keep your eyes peeled!"

Autism experiences vary along a spectrum in areas such as:

- Sensitivity to sensory experiences – being over- or under-sensitive to light, sound, taste, and touch
- Focus – intense focus on an area which could be a hobby, work, or interest; sometimes to the detriment of other life areas
- Communication – some people are unable to speak, some are limited, whilst others have good language skills but might struggle to pick up on tone of voice changes. As Sarah described, some can take things literally and need extra time to process information in some forms. Understanding others and the unwritten rules of the social world can be a challenge
- Repetitive behaviours – 'stimming' is the word used to describe repetitive or unusual movement or noises such as hand flapping, finger flicking, and rocking, which are often used to cope with a challenging situation
- Routine – needing a stable routine and finding sudden changes of plan overwhelming

If you want to learn more about autism, Sarah recommends speaking to an autistic person, finding communities on social media, or looking on the National Autistic Society website.[30]

ADHD (attention deficit hyperactivity disorder) is where there are persistent patterns of difficulties with attention and/or hyperactivity and impulsivity that interfere with day-to-day functioning.

The ADHD Foundation offers advice and support.[31]

---

[30] https://www.autism.org.uk/

[31] https://www.adhdfoundation.org.uk/

Personality characteristics

Personality is a description of how we think, feel, and behave, and offers another way to understand yourself.

We are born with a temperament, which you can see in babies as soon as they arrive in the world. Experiences with people around us interact with this temperament and shape who we are.

Personality frameworks are often used to help categorise our patterns, and they describe continuums such as extraversion at one end and introversion at the other. These can be helpful if we acknowledge that although there might be characteristics that we are more comfortable showing than others, we can draw on all parts of the continuum.

How we think, feel, and behave is also dependent on who we are with, and the situation we are in. How do I think, feel, and behave with this person/group in this context? If you feel comfortable with someone, and in a familiar setting, you might feel relaxed, confident, and outgoing. Conversely, with someone you have just met in a totally alien environment, the opposite might be true.

Personality is played out through relationships, so how we behave is often driven by a need to feel safe, loved, and be seen to be good at something. It is argued that being able to flex the characteristics you show (depending on the situation) helps improve performance and wellbeing. If something matters to us – such as striving for a goal – this can make it easier. If you have characteristics that feel very comfortable to you, and are in an established pattern, acting in ways opposite to this can be uncomfortable.

The 'Big 5' personality characteristics are the most established descriptions of personality (see the following table). There is no characteristic that is better than others – they all have strengths and downsides depending on the situation. *Which ones do you recognise as characteristics you are more comfortable showing?* How 'we are' can change under pressure and stress, so we will explore this and how to manage it effectively in Chapter 5.

The Big 5 personality characteristics

Low	High
Openness to experience	
Likes familiarity Likes certainty	Likes to try new things Enjoys change Optimistic
Conscientiousness	
Flexible and spontaneous Goes with the flow Lives in the moment	Hard-working Organised Follows rules
Extraversion	
Needs time to process their own thoughts Needs time alone to recharge	Outgoing Gets energy from being with others
Agreeableness	
Can be direct with others Focused on getting things done rather than keeping people happy	Likes to please others Wants to keep the peace and avoid conflict
Neuroticism	
Appears calm Doesn't often express emotions	Shows emotions readily under stress

Feedback from others about how they see you can help you develop insight and awareness. Asking for feedback, using the Big 5 characteristics above, can make this seem less daunting. Remember that how you come across to someone else illustrates how they view the world and the impact it has on them. We will explore this in more detail in Chapter 4 on relationships.

Athlete personality characteristics

A high-performance sport environment can encourage or attract people with certain characteristics. Extremes of any characteristic might be helpful in achieving goals but can result in unhelpful consequences along the way. The important thing is to be self-aware and recognise which characteristics are serving you. With awareness and reflection, you are more likely to be able to make a conscious choice, weighing up benefits and costs.

Let's explore those commonly thought to be important for athlete success.

Conscientiousness – if you are high in this characteristic, you would be hardworking, organised, and diligent. It is possible to show some parts of this trait but not others. I know athletes who are hardworking and committed to training, but their life administration is chaos (putting it politely)! This can be frustrating to those around them but doesn't impact on their ability to perform.

The ability to commit and work hard in training seems to be the common factor amongst high-performing athletes. Many athletes said they were able to work hard at their sport but not at other things that didn't interest them or matter.

Perfectionism – this term refers to someone who refuses to accept anything short of perfection, which is often an unrealistic or undefined standard. Perceived failure to reach this standard can cause distress.

There are three types of perfectionism:
1. Self-oriented where you expect yourself to be perfect
2. Other-oriented, where you expect others to be perfect
3. Socially-prescribed perfectionism, where you feel others expect you to be perfect

Self-oriented perfectionism has been linked to a drive to achieve goals but also to feeling anxious if you don't feel you have met the standard you want. It can lead to burnout if the drive to achieve is not balanced with recovery.

A healthy approach focuses on being the best you can be *under the circumstances*, rather than purely on an outcome or standard. You can do this by having a checklist of things in your control in areas that influence the outcome. It can be hard to be objective about whether you have done your best, as we can be overly critical of ourselves, so having someone else to discuss this with is critical.

The reality is that perfection is hard to define, and athletes who perform at their best on the day of competition can still make mistakes and do well.

Other-oriented perfectionism can create problems in relationships if your expectations are not realistic or not communicated in a healthy way.

Socially-prescribed perfectionism has been linked to feelings of depression and hopelessness if you feel you are not living up to the expectations of others. This could be real or perceived expectation. It is normal to care what others think about you, but not to the extent it causes you distress. We will explore how to manage this in Chapter 4, which is about relationships.

Obsession – this is when something continually preoccupies your mind, making it hard to think of anything else, and it often drives behaviours that support what you are obsessed with. It is easy to see why this characteristic is often seen in athletes, especially if it is their full-time job. If you want to be the best you can be, focus on the details that matter.

Some athletes I spoke to described themselves as obsessed, whilst others preferred to use the word passionate. Matt Walker, a downhill mountain biker, said, "You must love what you do as it takes hard work. For me, obsession means you can't do anything else, and you rely on it too much, which is unhealthy." Annie Last, a cross country mountain biker, said, "You have to be 100% committed and want it, but if you are obsessed you might make emotional rather than rational decisions, which could result in injury or burnout." Lutalo Muhammad looks at balance over a long period of time, "There are times when there is imbalance, and you have a single focus, but you need to know when to take time off and take your foot off the gas. That will be different for everyone. A perfect balance – always – is unrealistic. I like to read as a way of switching off from sport."

We have seen that if only one thing matters in life, that can have unhelpful consequences, especially if that area is not going well. Keeping some perspective and being able to switch on and off when you need to can help to mitigate against unhelpful obsession. It goes back to making a conscious choice, having weighed it all up. There might be times in your life when you want to obsessively focus on something and are happy to accept what goes with that.

Selfishness – this is defined as lacking consideration for other people and being focused on yourself. A study of GB athletes[32] who have won multiple medals found many reported putting greater importance on achievement compared to being nice or liked and recognised.

Whilst selfishness isn't a desirable characteristic in everyday life, it could be helpful in a sporting setting. Athletes I spoke to said you can make decisions that help your performance but also communicate in a way that shows consideration for others. For example, you might not go on a night out, but you can explain to those around you why you are doing this, and when you will be able to see them.

Keely Hodgkinson said, "It is about being able to switch to being all about you *when it matters*. I was at a competition doing my pre-race warm-up when a coach asked for a picture. Any other time I am happy to do this, but I had to say no as it would have impacted my preparation."

Athletes that can focus on themselves in a way that maintains positive relationships with those around them are more likely to be happier overall. As we saw in the meaning section, earlier in this chapter, focusing on others – not just yourself – is good for your mental health.

Resilience – The term resilience has been increasingly used in recent times and it refers to the ability to use personal qualities to withstand pressure. You can maintain functioning and

---

[32] Hardy, L. *et al.* (2017) Great British Medallists: Psychological biographies of super elite and elite athletes from Olympic Sports. *Progress in Brain Research.*

performance when under pressure and bounce back from challenges.

It is not a fixed trait that you have or don't have; it can change over time, it can be developed, and can be influenced by the environment and circumstances you are in. Being resilient doesn't mean you don't feel or show emotions; in fact, learning to recognise and process your emotions helps you build it up. It is not 'being tough' or not showing vulnerability (for example, playing through injury or saying you feel ok when you don't).

Personal characteristics such as optimism and conscientiousness are linked to resilience. No matter how resilient you are at any point in time, if a certain combination of factors arise, you might struggle. This is not a weakness, just a reality that – as humans – we all have limits to what we can deal with.

Developing flexibility in your personality characteristics

Being able to show a range of characteristics to suit the person or situation is a helpful skill to develop. This doesn't mean changing who you are, or not being true to yourself, but being able to dial aspects up or down to help you achieve a goal or develop a relationship.

Take introversion, for example. Some athletes feel most comfortable with people they know well and like to have time by themselves to recharge. If you are part of a team, or sharing a room on trips, this can be difficult. Being aware of this need, finding ways to get time by yourself, but also pushing yourself out of your comfort zone to develop relationships is a good way to develop flexibility.

One athlete explained, "I would describe myself as an introvert. I am encouraging myself to talk to people I don't know as well, and find it easier to ask them questions about themselves to get a conversation going. If I am sharing a room, we have a chat about time to ourselves, such as just before bed. This makes it less awkward if I put my headphones in and don't talk for a while."

Finding a reason why you want to develop a characteristic is a good starting point (for example, becoming more organised, so you don't leave an essential piece of equipment behind; or being more assertive, so others do not take advantage of you). Asking someone who shows the characteristic you want to improve how they do it can give you good ideas to try out.

Improving skills related to resilience has been shown to improve mental health and wellbeing.[33] One aspect is to explore what you see as pressure and threatening versus an opportunity or a challenge. Developing a mindset where you see situations as challenges to embrace helps with this. Being able to acknowledge and manage fears and worries is another skill to develop (see Chapter 5).

As discussed previously, having an environment and a coach that gets the balance of challenge and support right will help you be resilient. The impact of relationships on resilience is huge and will be discussed in Chapter 4. Practising performing when there is a consequence and gradually increasing the challenge can help develop resilience. This might include simulating a competition environment by inviting in competitors, setting time limits, or having distractions.

Happiness

When we think about how we want to be, we often say, 'I want to be happy.' This is an understandable desire, but we are generally not good at predicting what will lead to feelings of happiness or accepting that happiness is a transient state.

Understanding how we experience pleasure is a good place to start, as it is not how you might expect.

Pleasure and pain are linked in the brain.[34] Imagine a see-saw with pleasure at one end and pain and discomfort at the other. When we experience something that is pleasurable, that side of the see-saw tips down and we get a dopamine release. The brain wants to

---

[33] Sarkar, M. & Page, A. E. (2022) Developing individual and team resilience in elite sport: research into practice, *Journal of Sport Psychology in Action*.

[34] *Dopamine nation: finding balance in the age of indulgence.* Dr Anna Lembke (2021)

maintain balance, however, so to bring the see-saw back down, it tips over to the pain side in an equal and oppositive way first. Therefore, a feeling of pleasure and happiness doesn't last that long. You have just watched an episode of your favourite Netflix series and the good feeling quickly goes. You want to feel good again, so you watch another, then another! The more we press on the pleasure side with instant sources of pleasure, the more we need to feel the same good feeling.

Quick releases of dopamine can come from things like social media, video games, alcohol, etc. Healthier ways to get pleasure include time outside in nature, and spending time with people you love. Sadly, the more time we spend doing the quick-fix things, the less we enjoy or seek out these other activities. We can check how much we are relying on instant sources of pleasure, and put measures in place to avoid using them to excess (e.g., by having a break or limiting use). It is easy to use things such as social media in a way that doesn't help us feel good in the long term, so experiment to see what works for you.

The see-saw effect happens in the other direction as well; when you do something hard or uncomfortable, you feel good afterwards. Choosing to do things that are challenging is therefore good for us and provides a healthier route to dopamine. These include things such as a tough training session, cold showers, and behaving or thinking in ways out of your comfort zone.

Inevitably, many people experience pain from difficult things that happen in their lives, so that side of the see-saw is already being pressed. It is understandable that – to cope with this – we often reach for those instant ways to feel better, even if they don't last long. The aim of therapy is to help people cope with and work through their pain in ways that are helpful in the longer term.

How the brain balances pleasure and pain helps us understand why the reward we get from winning can be fleeting. When we reach a goal, dopamine levels rise and then plummet. Athletes often say that they thought the happiness from reaching their goals would last longer than it did, and instead, they can feel down.

After winning gold at her first Olympic Games in 2012, when she was just 19 years old, Jade Jones said she struggled. "I loved the feeling of winning, but soon afterwards I felt lost. It is something

I had dreamed of since being a kid, and now I had done it. I thought I would be happy forever, but I wasn't."

If we recognise and expect this, we can reward ourselves for doing the hard things on the journey to our goals and not just focus on achieving the goal, which is not guaranteed. We can learn to enjoy the process of working hard, which will increase the chances of the outcome we want. Tell yourself you like the tough sessions!

Our expectations also have an impact on the pleasure we experience. If something good happens that you didn't expect, you typically feel great. If you expect it and it then happens, you get an increase in pleasure whilst anticipating it, then a small amount when you get it. Expecting something good that doesn't happen brings about a drop in dopamine below baseline, which is the feeling of disappointment. This could be why the bronze medallist who didn't expect to be on the podium seems happier than the silver medallist who expected gold.

Comparison can also impact on how happy we feel. We are more likely to compare ourselves to those who have more rather than less. In doing so, we fail to appreciate what we have or how far we have come. We get used to the good things in our life over time and can take them for granted. Writing a gratitude journal once a week has been shown to help bring them back into our conscious thoughts.

Studies have found that people think things such as money or possessions will make them happy, but we quickly get used to what we have. Experiences and good quality relationships give much more satisfaction. Small acts of kindness towards others are another piece of the happiness puzzle. Even talking to strangers, such as the barista in the coffee shop, increases the feeling of social connection and helps us feel good.

Having meaning and purpose has been found to result in happiness as a by-product; actively seeking happiness, by comparison, often backfires.

> *Activity*
>
> Write down how you want to be. How do you want to think, feel, and behave? You might include your mental health definition from Chapter 1 as well as characteristics such as positive, calm, kind, fun, determined. There are no right or wrong answers. Which ones would you like to develop, and which come more naturally to you? You can be curious and reflect on the patterns you have that help or make this harder.
>
> Write down one action you can take to move you in the direction you want to go.

Summary

How we think, feel, and behave is influenced by:

- The temperament we are born with
- Relationships with caregivers and life experiences
- Beliefs that shape how we see ourselves, the world, and how we relate to others (including our values, meaning, and self-worth)
- What is happening in our body and the sense we make of it
- The person or group we are with
- The situation we are in
- By understanding that the brain's job is to keep us alive – and how it makes predictions based on past experiences and beliefs – we can become more aware of our automatic patterns and take steps to change them if we want to
- Happiness doesn't come from where you might expect; it comes from having meaning and purpose outside of yourself and healthy connections with others
- Developing self-awareness through regular reflection and taking time to work out *your* values, meaning, identity, and where *you* get your self-worth from will increase your wellbeing

- Develop a sense of self-worth from your personal characteristics, not just achieving outcomes. Reward yourself for, and get enjoyment from, the effort and experience along the way
- Changing patterns can be hard as they helped serve a purpose at some point in our lives, but it is worth the effort to live the life you want to

To improve wellbeing, you can:

- Explore your values (what is important to you in life)
- Create meaning (through belonging, having a purpose outside of yourself and the story you tell about your life experiences). Doing things that are meaningful to you helps you get through tough times
- Look at where you get your self-worth from, and explore if this is helpful
- Develop more than one identity in your life

Understand the brain better:

- Every brain is unique, with its job being to keep you alive and well. Understanding *your* brain can help you navigate the world more effectively
- Your brain makes predictions automatically, based on experience, knowledge, and beliefs. These predictions influence the thoughts and feeling you have and are not always accurate or helpful so are worth examining

Personality is important:

- Personality continuums are another way to understand yourself
- Our personalities are influenced by who we are with, and the situation we are in
- We can reflect on which parts help or hinder living the life we want, and work on developing flexibility in the characteristics we show

Chapter 4: Relationships

- How important are relationships for our mental health?
- How do we form relationships, and how can we improve them?
- What are healthy and unhealthy relationships?
- How can we manage difficult conversations effectively?
- How can we cope with the loss of a relationship?

How important are relationships for our mental health?

Relationships can be the best *and* worst thing for our mental health. Life involves other people, so it is impossible to consider mental health without examining relationships.

Good quality relationships help us cope better with the challenges of life, bring us joy, and give us a sense of belonging. We can tolerate pain and recover quicker when supported by loved ones. Spending time with people you feel a connection with can lower the levels of cortisol (a stress hormone) in your body. Other people can help us manage our emotions, problem-solve, and open the door to new opportunities.

Loneliness, on the other hand, has been linked to mental and physical issues and is said to be as bad for you as smoking 15 a day. Loneliness is when you want social interaction, but you don't have the amount you would like. This is different to those who like time by themselves and do this by choice.

The Covid 19 pandemic highlighted the importance of social connection and how hard it can be if you can't see other people. If you are struggling mentally, you might not want to interact with people as much as you usually do, which exacerbates the problem. Finding ways to keep connected with others during these times is critical and is an important aspect of preventing and managing mental difficulties.

The key here is *healthy relationships*. If you have experienced challenging relationships, you will know the negative impact these can have. It is important to know what a healthy relationship is and how to deal with an unhealthy one. Some of us find relationships easier than others, but all of us will have times when we find them emotionally tricky. Let's look at how we learnt how to interact with others, and how this influences our relationships today. We will go back to your first relationship… with your parents or main caregiver.

How we form relationships

Imagine when you were a newborn baby; you were totally dependent on those around you to keep you alive and well. Even before you were born, you were able to pick up on the emotional state of your mother. These experiences, along with the first few years of your life, have direct and enduring impacts on how your brain develops.

In the early years, you must form a bond with the person caring for you and be able to communicate your needs without language, and – as you develop – you need to feel safe and secure, show a range of emotions, learn how to handle these emotions, and feel understood. You can't do this on your own. You and the caregiver must tune into each other's minds and bodies, and this is done through facial expressions, tone of voice, and touch.

You will influence each other at a physiological level, changing heart rate, breathing, and blood pressure. Ideally, the person looking after you can be consistent, emotionally available, and empathic – helping to reassure and calm you when you need it as well as encouraging play and excitement.

As you get older, they need to help you manage frustration and set boundaries. Having feelings ignored or denied ("Don't be silly, you don't feel scared") can impact on how we feel in the future. If they are denied, they don't disappear. We need to learn that – whatever emotions we experience – we are still worthy, and however bad we feel, it will pass. There is someone there who can accept how we feel and not be overwhelmed. This emotional need remains in adult life.

How others respond to your emotional states and needs, and help you regulate them, paves the way for how *you* manage social relationships. It helps you form bonds with others, understand how you are both feeling, and read social situations. It helps you recognise and tolerate your own emotions and behave in a helpful manner (this is called self-regulation). This can be carried out in two ways:

1. *Interactive regulation* – choosing to go to another person to help manage your internal states, to share feelings, and get comfort
2. *Auto-regulation* – Using your own resources to soothe or calm yourself

One is not better than the other, and we need to develop the flexibility to do both. Parents and caregivers are typically trying their best and might be dealing with their own mental struggles whilst providing care. This means they won't be completely present or always tuned into the child. They might feel anxious and find it hard to give reassurance. They might get the level of challenge wrong, so the child feels shame. This is normal in any relationship; it is how often it happens and how it is repaired that matters.

Sadly, some early life experiences involve abuse or neglect. This impacts on how that person deals with their own and others' emotions and can impact on their ability to build trust. It can also impact on their physiology. During periods of abuse, the brain detects threats and can remain in a constant state of readiness, altering the production of hormones such as cortisol and adrenaline, which takes its toll on the body and mind. Understandably, this shapes how they see the world; it is not a safe place where people can be trusted. They are on high alert even when the threat has gone. Experiencing such trauma is a painful thing to endure, and no one should ever have to experience this. With support, it is possible to manage this pain and develop healthy connections.

How you interact with people in your current relationships is, therefore, a product of previous interactions and unconscious patterns you have developed. Emotional difficulties are often rooted in these relationship patterns. Below are some common patterns called *attachment styles*. You might recognise all of them, depending on the person you are with or situation you are in… or there might be one that stands out. It is likely that many of us are not securely attached at all times; this is the reality of being a human raised by other humans. Awareness is the first step in helping you to determine if the patterns are helpful or not. Which of these can you relate to?

Attachment style patterns

Secure

This pattern sees the world as safe and predictable. You can form close relationships and be vulnerable with others. You believe you are worthy of love. You can set boundaries in relationships, communicate your needs, and think conflicts can be resolved. You balance independence with closeness to others and can empathise effectively. You can regulate by yourself and with others. You tend to trust readily.

Avoidant

This style has difficulty believing emotional needs can be met by others. Emotions are not understood, so there is no point showing them. You can find it hard to be vulnerable with others which can make committing to a relationship difficult. It can be hard to recognise your own and others' emotions and you might seem distant. You are less likely to ask for support if you are finding things hard and might withdraw to try and self-soothe (sometimes using distractions such as training, technology, or substances rather than acknowledging feelings).

You value thinking and logic over feelings and often want practical advice rather than support. You might find it hard when others show vulnerability or distress. It is hard for others to tell if you are struggling until you suddenly break down, often when something important to you is not going well. You might seem independent or mature for your age. Sporting environments often encourage avoidant behaviour such as being strong mentally and physically, avoiding showing weakness or talking about how you feel.

Anxious

This pattern fears being abandoned and being disconnected from others. This is an understandable human fear that we all have (to some degree) as we need other people to survive. This can lead to feeling insecure and wanting to test out how someone else feels about you. This might come across as needy, but you are seeking reassurance and connection.

You can find it hard to be on your own or out of a relationship, and often want to commit early on. Fear of being rejected can lead to intense emotions. Thinking about how the relationship is going can take up a lot of mental energy, and you might feel dissatisfied. You might want others to help soothe and regulate your emotions. To avoid rejection, you might show people-pleasing behaviours and find it hard to say no or set boundaries.

Here are some ideas for improving relationships based on the patterns you recognise in yourself and others. This might be something you want to explore with someone you trust, or a professional, especially if this feels difficult to think about.

Yourself – Avoidant

- Reflect on why you might not want to share how you feel or who you are; for example, not wanting to feel judged or feeling you should be able to solve problems yourself. Are these beliefs accurate and helpful in your life now?
- Would there be any benefits in letting someone know how you are feeling, or revealing something about yourself?
- Notice what someone else does that leads you to withdraw or close off. Start paying attention to your internal bodily signs like heart rate and breathing and link them to feelings. Develop your ability to describe how you feel, rather than how you think, by using the feelings wheel[35]
- Recognise when you go to facts and logic or avoid a subject rather than acknowledging or saying how you feel
- If you want to feel in control, recognising and expressing feelings regularly helps prevent a big outburst or breakdown where you might lose control
- By writing down or voicing your worries and fears 'out loud', you are in a better place to manage them. Ignoring them doesn't make them go away

---

[35] https://blog.calm.com/blog/the-feelings-wheel

- If someone is showing vulnerability or distress, see if you can sit with them and listen, even if you want to leave the situation or you feel uncomfortable

Others – Avoidant

- Just because others don't show emotions doesn't mean they don't have them
- Model being vulnerable and showing how you feel (this is powerful if this is someone an individual respects, such as their coach)
- Help them develop an emotional vocabulary
- Ask 'How are you really doing?' or 'I was wondering if you are feeling ....' or 'I guess when you say you are fine, you might be worrying about the game at the weekend; I know I have felt like that'
- Talk side-by-side, or on a walk, as this feels less intense
- Listen out for passing comments that show how they are feeling
- It can take a long time before someone talks about how they feel, so be patient
- Give them space and don't see not wanting to talk as rejection
- Emotions might be expressed through actions not words (such as doing something practical to show they care)

Yourself – Anxious

- To improve self-regulation, you can get support from someone you find reassuring and who will help problem-solve. They can help you recognise and reflect on the feelings you are having, explore why, and then help you manage them. You can then start to use the same strategies yourself. Learning breathing exercises such as box breathing (in through your nose for a count of 4, hold for 4, out for 4, hold for 4, and repeat) can also help with intense emotions
- Explore your fears, such as rejection or criticism. This is your mind trying to help you survive, but fear can drive behaviours that move us away from what we want. Go

from guessing what someone else is thinking to asking them or considering other thoughts. Writing down your worries can help you work out if there is any truth in them or not. The ideas in Chapter 5 about managing fear and anxiety can help you with this
- You are likely to find a relationship with someone showing secure rather than avoidant patterns easier to manage. An anxious and avoidant combination can result in an increasing need for closeness, which pushes the avoidant person further away. There will be less drama in a relationship with a secure style, which might seem unexciting at first

Others – Anxious

- Others might not ask for help, but being upset is a signal they want support
- Show you have heard and understood how they are feeling before trying to reassure them
- Be consistent and do what you say you will do
- Set boundaries early in the relationship, so they know what to expect from you
- Regular, small reassurances can go a long way
- Help them manage their feelings by being calm yourself, and gradually encourage them to understand their emotions and problem-solving. Don't get sucked into the intense emotions

---

Activity

Which of the above patterns do you recognise in your relationships? Think about how you communicate remotely as well as face-to-face. Which of the ideas could you try?

Improving relationships

A good relationship doesn't mean that you always agree, and everything is rosy. It does mean that you feel respected. By focusing on the following elements, and practising these skills, you can make improvements in your current relationships. This checklist applies to all types of relationship.

Listening, understanding, and empathising

We like to think we are good listeners, but listening is hard to do well. By listening and showing you have understood someone, you are demonstrating they matter.

All humans want to feel seen and understood, but due to distractions and our own thoughts, we don't always provide this.

Being fully present with someone is the *best way* to build a connection. How often are you half-listening or waiting to get your point across? How often do you ignore a sign that they want your attention? To listen effectively, we need to focus on what others are saying, ask questions, put aside assumptions, and manage the noise in our own heads. We need to show them we have understood how they are thinking and feeling and remember it in future conversations. Technology has undoubtedly made this harder. Think how often you are with someone but not present as you scroll away on your phone.

To understand others better, we need to acknowledge that we all have unique brains and see the world differently. They might have different values, personality characteristics, life experiences, knowledge, or be neurodivergent (such as autistic, ADHD, dyslexic). This quote is one person's experience of being autistic: "Everyone around me has a disorder which makes them say things they don't mean, not care about structure, fail to hyperfocus on singular important topics, have unreliable memories, drop weird hints, and creepily stare into my eyeballs. So why do people say I am the weird one? Because there's more of them than me." [36]

Autistic people can have varying degrees of empathy – the same as non-autistic people – and experience emotions, although some struggle to identify or show emotions, which might come across as distant. Unwritten social rules can be confusing, so be aware of this. Autistic people can suppress behaviours and learn how to

---

[36] www.autisticnotweird.com

show socially accepted ones, which is called *masking*. This can be tiring and difficult for long periods of time.

ADHD can mean someone finds it hard to listen and gets distracted easily. Understanding the teenage brain is also helpful here. Our brains are not fully developed until around 25 years of age, and during the teenage years, we are developing the ability to manage impulses and make decisions with the future in mind. Peer relationships become increasingly important, and some teenagers take more risks and test the limits when in the presence of friends. The drive to fit in can lead to decisions that make sense in the moment, but don't always fit in with longer-term goals.

Empathy helps relationships. To really understand someone, you need to be able to see things from their point of view, even if it is not how you would see it. *Emotional empathy* is when we share emotional experiences and our heart rate and breathing synchronises. This could happen if we are sharing experiences like watching sport, music, comedy, or dancing together. It is a powerful way to bond to feel the same emotion at the same time.

Other emotions like sadness can be shared, "My friend told me about the loss of their dog who had been part of the family for 15 years. I felt sadness and tears in my eyes as they told me about it."

Cognitive empathy is being able to show someone you understand how they think and feel without experiencing those feelings yourself. You can imagine what it would be like to be in their shoes. If you had the same view of the world that they did, how would you feel?

Compassionate empathy moves beyond understanding how they feel to taking action to support them. This might be sitting with them and showing you can handle their emotions without distracting them or denying them, helping them feel safe, offering advice, or practical support like cooking them dinner. Often, people want to vent and don't want advice. Notice how often you rush to tell them what to do or dismiss their feelings ("come on, don't feel like that"). Always validate their feelings first.

Balance of appreciation to criticism

Relationships that have a higher ratio of criticism to appreciation can feel difficult. Even in a coach-athlete relationship – where you *want* feedback – if all you hear is criticism, it can impact negatively on the relationship. Think about how often *you* tell someone that you appreciate them and how much *you* criticise them.

Expressing needs and respecting boundaries

A healthy relationship means you can be honest about what you need and what you don't want. This is called *setting boundaries*.

Boundaries have been described as "The distance at which I can love you and me at the same time".[37] If you keep people too far away, and have too strict boundaries, you won't be able to connect with them; if you let people behave how they want, you can lose the love and respect for yourself.

Having self-worth makes it easier to set boundaries. In the context of relationships, this might involve how much time alone or together you need, how you want to communicate (length of time to respond to messages and calls, acceptable tone of voice), and what behaviours are acceptable. If you find yourself saying yes to things that you don't want to do, or tolerating behaviour you know is wrong, you might need to look at your boundaries. If you are worried about pleasing someone, this can make it hard (the difficult conversations section will give you ideas about how to manage this).

Sometimes, you can make sacrifices for other people, or do things you don't want to, as you know it will make them happy, but this should be because it is a choice, not out of fear. In the athlete-coach relationship, boundaries might be about agreeing when you will message each other, when you will debrief, who makes what decision, etc. If one person is messaging late at night or too often, and this isn't helpful for the other person, setting a boundary would mean discussing this and agreeing to a new way of working.

Trust and honesty

You do what you say you will do, and don't share information about others without their permission. That is the simplest way to build trust. Honesty has a social element to it where we tread the line between politeness and brutal honesty, depending on the

---

[37] A quote from the therapist Prentis Hemphill.

situation. Some people want things sugar-coated, others do not(!), so it is good to find out. If withholding the information would harm or upset the person if they found out, then honesty is the right thing. Autistic people can take honesty literally, which can be seen as blunt; rather than asking them to 'be honest with you', you might need to give them some guidance.

Shared goals

Not all relationships will have this, but a shared goal is a good way to develop a connection. You support each other to work towards the goal. In team situations, this might be the only thing you have in common; you don't have to like someone to develop this element of your relationship.

Sharing the highs and lows of life

Meaningful relationships can share both fun and hard times. If someone disappears when things are not going well, or you are not winning, this tells you a lot about that relationship.

You want the best for each other

You should want them to be happy and support them to grow and develop. This can be tricky for team sport athletes as someone else developing could mean they take your spot. Seeing it as an opportunity to learn from them and be inspired to develop yourself can help.

You can accept each other and be yourself

Wanting to change someone is not a good basis for a relationship. You can give them feedback on the impact they are having, but ultimately it is their choice to change or not; you then must decide what you want to do if they don't want to change. There is a difference between accepting someone's personality quirks and accepting bad behaviour. If you are constantly frustrated with someone, and you know they don't want to change, you have not fully accepted them. You should feel like you can be yourself and be accepted. Trying to be someone you are not takes effort and prevents genuine connection.

You can work through disagreements and mistakes

It is normal to disagree, make a mistake, misunderstand, or inadvertently hurt someone. It is how we avoid making the same mistake or having the same disagreement in the future that matters. You can repair the relationship by saying sorry and acknowledging the role you played. You should be able to work through disagreements without attacking the other person.

Interdependence not dependence

As was discussed in the secure attachment section, being able to balance independence with closeness is important. You don't rely on one person to fulfil all your needs, and you are not completely dependent on them.

Equitable

The relationship feels fair, with both people able to share decisions. There is agreement on splitting things like time, tasks, and money. It doesn't have to be equal, but both sides must be happy.

> *Activity*
>
> Which of the elements listed above come naturally to you, and which take more work?
>
> Think about a relationship you would like to improve. Write down the actions you can take. Think about your personality characteristics from Chapter 3. Which ones will help, and which ones might you need to dial up or down?

Unhealthy relationships

Unhealthy relationships exist on a spectrum, ranging from uncomfortable tension to abusive. If you have grown up surrounded by unhealthy behaviours, some of these might seem normal and acceptable, and it is harder to tell if someone has crossed the line. Talking to someone else you trust will help you work out if they are unacceptable behaviours. You can talk to a safeguarding person in your club or national governing body or the advice lines below.[38] Abuse includes physical, psychological, and sexual abuse, as well as neglect (failure to meet physical and emotional needs, or failure to protect from harm). Sometimes, we can make excuses for bad behaviour or see it as an act of caring or love. If someone is struggling mentally, they might not behave like their usual self, but poor mental health is never an excuse for abusive behaviour.

Coercive control

The aim of this behaviour is to isolate you from others, exploit you, or take away independence and control. This could include controlling who you see, where you go, your social media, your money, and using put-downs and humiliation to make you feel worthless or unsafe. Thankfully, this is now a criminal offence.

You might have heard the term *gaslighting*; this is the use of coercion to make you doubt your experiences and memories. An example might be having a view about the other person constantly being late. The gaslighter might say, "You have a weird view on timekeeping, and there is something wrong with you for thinking that way", rather than accepting your point. They might manipulate you into thinking you did something and then forgot. Our memories are not perfect, so they play on this to confuse and control. These can be subtle rather than overt behaviours.

Tries to change the other person

This behaviour is also linked to control. They don't accept who you are and want you to change how you dress, speak, or your interests. This criticism can chip away at your confidence and make you question your identity. Another way someone can try to change a person is by becoming a *rescuer*. They decide that they can help someone with their struggles and know what is best for them. They get their self-worth from being needed and taking care of

---

[38] Refuge domestic abuse helpline for women 0800 2000 247 | Men's Advice Line 0808 8010 327
https://www.nhs.uk/live-well/healthy-body/getting-help-for-domestic-violence/ For advice and further information on the signs of emotional, physical, and sexual abuse.

someone else. They might put up with bad behaviour as they believe they can change an individual once they have fixed them.

Lack of trust

If you trust someone, you won't feel the need to control or question them. Jealousy springs from a lack of trust.

Makes threats

Making threats is a way to manipulate or control someone even if the threats are not carried out. This could be threats of physical harm, withholding resources, or unwanted outcomes.

Doesn't respect boundaries, opinions, and feelings

If you have told someone what is acceptable and they ignore it, or they ask you to do something you are not comfortable with, they are not respecting your boundaries. You should be able to have an opinion, even if the other person doesn't agree with it. You should be able to disagree and have a discussion. Contempt is when you disregard someone's feelings and treat them as worthless, and it is the *number one predictor* of relationships ending. This can take the form of hostile humour, sneering and eye-rolling, and people communicating they think they are better than you.

Avoiding difficult topics or using the silent treatment

It is understandable that we don't always feel ready or able to talk about difficult topics. However, constantly avoiding them, or completely refusing to talk at all (sometimes for days at a time), is not healthy and damages the connection.

Blaming

All the responsibility for difficulties in the relationship is put on the other person with no acknowledgement of the part that the blamer has played. This often leads to the other person feeling attacked and becoming defensive.

If you recognise any of these actions in your relationships, talk to someone you trust or use the helplines.

Athlete and coach relationship

The relationship with your coach is so important; it can impact on how much you enjoy sport and how much you develop as a person and athlete. The elements of a healthy relationship are just as important in the athlete-coach relationship as any other, especially with the power that the coach role has. A positive coach-athlete relationship should enable you to perform at your best and be mentally healthy. Coaching is a role with a huge level of responsibility. It is often after an athlete retires and starts coaching that they appreciate how tough the coach role is!

Let's look at two aspects of this relationship that can cause issues if not managed well.

Control/decision making

Most humans have a need for some degree of control in their lives and without it, we can feel helpless or unmotivated. There are three approaches that can be used:

1. Coach-centred – the athlete follows instructions from the coach
2. Coach-athlete-centred – there is give and take and collaboration between athlete and coach
3. Athlete-centred – the athlete makes the decisions

With the *coach-centred approach*, you could have an athlete that is happy to defer all decisions and planning to the coach as they trust them and their experience. They don't want to know the ins and outs of decisions and are happy to follow a plan. On the other hand, you can have an athlete that would like more involvement but isn't given the option, causing friction. This approach can foster dependence where the athlete can't perform or make decisions if the coach isn't telling them what to do. This might be used if the coach has a lot of experience, and the athlete is younger or less experienced.

The coach should always be willing to explain *why* they have created the plan the way they have, and answer questions, as this will help with buy-in. There will be some decisions that a person in power will need to make. If athletes believe they have had their views heard and understood, and know the reasons why, they are more likely to be engaged.

The cyclist Chris Opie explained, "The coach was very good at letting us know which decisions we could get involved with and which he would make. He would explain the reasons for decisions so – even if we didn't always agree with them – it was easier to accept."

It is helpful to ask coaches what they are basing their decisions on in areas such as selection. If it is based on outcomes, you can focus your energy on the aspects that give you the best chance of achieving them. Behaviours such as commitment or supporting teammates might also play a part.

The *coach-athlete-centred approach* considers the thoughts and experiences of both parties when putting a plan together. Both parties jointly problem-solve, respecting each other's views. This approach might be more likely with an experienced or older athlete, or an athlete that doesn't respond well to being told what to do.

The *athlete-centred approach* is where the athlete drives planning and decision-making, asking for ideas or support if they need them. It is not always easy to get the balance right, especially in team sports where it is harder to consider everyone's opinions. It can feel scary for a coach to relinquish decisions or give athletes freedom, but ultimately it is the athlete's life and career, and they should be able to ask questions and be involved.

Paula Dunn, UK Athletics team leader, describes her approach, "If we are all there for the athlete to improve, your views shouldn't be that far apart. They can take or leave that advice. It is their career. It lies with them to make those changes. You have got to have a relationship, so they know you are there to support them. We focus on the areas we agree on. We can't force people to do anything, and they won't buy in if forced. We focus on the process – not outcomes – and put our energy into those."

> *Activity*
>
> Which approach do you and your coach currently take? What could be improved?

Challenge and support

After organisations have undergone investigations for actions such as bullying, the pendulum can swing too far the other way, with coaches treading on eggshells and not wanting to push or challenge for fear of criticism. Sport at the top level is tough and physically demanding. If your goal is to be the best you can be, and test that in a competitive environment, then you will need feedback and honesty. A coach's job can be to encourage more growth than you thought possible and help you tackle the challenges thrown up on your journey. There is also a performance bar that coaches cannot move. The balance of challenge and support should help you face difficulties in a helpful way.

What it takes to get the best out of each athlete can vary dramatically; some report that they like to be pushed hard or get direct and tough feedback in a shouty fashion, whilst for others, this does not work and can be overwhelming. Some days, we can handle honesty better than others, depending on our mental state and tiredness. In an ideal world, every coach would be able to adapt their style to suit each athlete, but sadly we don't live in that world.

Building a good relationship with your coach and being able to give each other feedback will help to get the challenge and support balance right. This is not an easy thing to do, especially as a young athlete with an experienced coach, with strong characters, or when you don't get to choose the coach you work with. In a team sport, it can be hard for a coach to find a style that works for everyone, but if you are really struggling, *you need to let them know*. Using their power to instil fear, intimidate, or manipulate is never acceptable. You will find feedback ideas to help you tackle a conversation with your coach below.

Aspects of a healthy athlete-coach relationship have been found to include:

1. Focusing on *commitment* (I feel committed to them, I feel close, I feel like my sports career is promising with them)
2. *Closeness* (refers to the bond expressed through trust, respect, appreciation, and liking, and being honest about how things are going)

3. *Complementarity* (refers to cooperative and collaborative behaviours)

High levels on these areas are associated with greater satisfaction with performance and personal treatment, and higher levels of team cohesion.[39] The attachment styles of you and your coach will impact on how you feel in these areas; for example, if you are anxious and they are avoidant, it can feel less satisfying.

Andy Turner talked about his relationship with his coach Lloyd. "I met him when I was 19. He helped develop me as a person, and we shared highs and lows. He knew how to adapt to us as athletes; he knew the days I wasn't 100% and would change things to get the best out of me." Lutalo Muhammad believes honesty is the key to a good relationship with your coach. "You don't have to have similar personalities and be two peas in a pod, as long as you are honest and can accept each other for who you are."

Trevor Painter and Jenny Meadows coach several athletes in athletics, including Keely Hodgkinson, the 800m runner. "Relationships are key to our coaching. We make time to understand those we work with. We do the values exercise when we start working with someone as it helps us understand them better and adapt how we coach them."

Trevor said, "I had someone in the group who I thought was there to improve their performance, but they wanted to socialise. That helped me know how to interact with them. The balance of push and challenge will vary, and I encourage them to think for themselves and give me feedback. Not every athlete can be an Olympic medallist, but if I can help them be the 'best they can be', I am happy."

Thinking about your relationship with your coach, consider the aspects you are happy with and those you would like to improve. Coaches are not mind-readers, so this might involve having a conversation about how you can get the best out of each other.

---

[39] Jowett, S. & Chaundy, V. (2004) An investigation into the impact of coach leadership and coach–athlete relationship on group cohesion. *Group Dynamics: Theory, Research and Practice.*

Managing difficult conversations

A conversation might be difficult if:

- You are worried about the consequences
- You don't like the person or see things differently from them
- It is an emotionally-charged topic
- You are giving feedback

Firstly, acknowledge and address your worries. Consider how likely they are to happen, and then devise a plan that increases the chance of things going well (using the points below). Avoidance is a common tactic but is not helpful in the long term. Issues can get worse or emotions simmering below the surface come out in unhelpful ways. Avoidance can lead to passive aggression, where you indirectly show you are not happy. This might mean being stubborn, putting off doing something you have agreed to, or saying it in a jokey or sarcastic way. Think about the benefits for the relationship if you have the conversation.

Before the conversation:

- Write down your ideal outcome. Accept that you might not achieve it, but you can increase the chances by being prepared. You can also come up with an outcome that you both buy into, such as improving the relationship or agreeing on a decision
- Think about the part both of you have played in the situation, and be willing to say what you could have done differently
- What feelings are you likely to have when you speak to them? What things might they say or do that you will find difficult? You want to be able to express how you feel without getting overwhelmed. Writing it down or practising the conversation with someone else can help with this. Pre-empting likely scenarios will help you come across how you want to
- Ask someone who knows them well for advice on the best way to approach the conversation

- Get support to plan the conversation. This could be someone outside of sport
- Consider the best time and place. Often, conversations where you are side by side – such as driving or walking – feel more relaxed. Text messages can get misinterpreted, so meet face-to-face when possible
- What goals or values do you share? As an athlete, a shared goal might be getting the best out of you in training and competition. Focusing on these helps to find common ground
- Prepare the points you want to make. There is a difference between facts and opinions. A fact is proven to be true, whilst an opinion is personal and is based on how you see the world. Most conversations revolve around opinions that people state as facts
- Initiating a conversation is a moment of bravery. By messaging or asking for a meeting, you are committing to it

During the conversation:

- Share the outcome you would like if it will help the conversation. "I would like to chat to you about my training plan and how we can get the most out of the preparation before the competition". Be *specific* with requests
- Listen to understand. If you don't listen and show you have understood how they feel, progress will be harder. Accept their feelings even if they seem unreasonable to you; they feel how they feel. Their feelings will help you work out their beliefs. Check you have understood what they have said or are feeling
- Don't over-interpret body language. Everyone expresses emotions differently, so it is hard to accurately gauge. You only really know how someone is feeling if they are willing to tell you
- 'You and me versus the problem' not 'you versus me.' If you are trying to score points, it becomes about who is right and wrong, rather than jointly solving the problem.

If you can look at the problem as something you both want to solve, rather than making it a battle, you are much more likely to have a productive conversation. Relationships where you are trying to get one up on the other person harm the connection. Sport is competitive, so it is likely this approach could seep into conversations
- Use 'I' rather than 'you' statements. 'I felt like I didn't get a chance to share my thoughts on that decision; I would like to have input next time, please, as it helps me commit to the plan if I am involved' instead of 'You are so inconsiderate, why didn't you consult me?' Using 'I' feels less attacking, so they are less likely to want to defend or attack back. You are entitled to an opinion, even if the other person doesn't agree with it
- Focus on the benefits of your ideas for the shared goal
- Be aware of your tone of voice, level of calmness, and words. You can influence the other person with your demeanour. This is hard when you care about what you are discussing, but *rehearsing* beforehand will help. Emotive words or absolutes like *always* or *never* can inflame the situation
- Focus on slowing down your breathing to help you regulate your heart rate; this will help you to stay calm
- Take a minute to think or come back to the conversation later. Sometimes, we need time to process what the other person has said
- You could take in a notepad with reminders to help you focus

You can complete this table before the conversation to help you prepare.

Question	Answer
What is my ideal outcome?	
What goals or values do we both share?	

Question	Answer
What might I find difficult about this conversation?	
Who can help me prepare or practice?	
What will help me be how I want to be? What will help me listen?	
What are the main points and facts I want to get across?	

Receiving feedback

It is not always easy to receive feedback, but it is helpful to learn how to take it on board if you want to improve in sport. The person delivering it, how they do it, and whether you agree will influence how you receive it. If you trust them and know they have your best interests at heart – and share your dreams and goals – that can help you take it onboard. Feedback could be:

- Appreciation or sharing positive aspects of what you have done
- How you compare to a standard
- Your behaviour and mindset
- Coaching on how to improve

To help you understand, you can ask for examples, remembering that what someone shares will reveal what matters to them. If they say you need to be more committed in how you complete a drill, for example, you know that they see commitment as a key element of performance. Practise separating your worth as a person from feedback on behaviours or skills... you are not your result! Focus on things you can control, like effort.

If you know that a certain style of feedback works best for you, discuss this with your coach, as they might not be aware of it. This is not to downplay how hard initiating this conversation can feel, and it can take courage to do something you find difficult. Developing the skill of doing difficult things will transfer to the competition arena and to life. Likewise, you will already have some of these skills, so remember to use them in difficult conversations.

Loss

Loss is a sad reality of life. It could be a loss of a loved one who has passed away, or the end of a relationship. Following loss, it is understandable that we can struggle emotionally. Social rejection has been shown to have the same impact on the brain as physical pain, which is why being ghosted can be hard to deal with.

Each culture has its own customs, rituals, and ways of expressing grief, and this can change over time. My nan grew up in the 1920s in Birmingham and loved telling us stories about her childhood. She said following the death of a loved one, it was common to wear black for up to a year.

Grief is the price we pay for love. You might have heard this phrase before; it comes from a book by the psychiatrist Dr Colin Murray. He says, "The pain of grief is just as much part of life as the joy of love: it is perhaps the price we pay for love, the cost of commitment. To ignore this fact, or to pretend that it is not so, is to put on emotional blinkers which leave us unprepared for the losses that will inevitably occur in our own lives."[40] He found that most people pass through four stages following loss, and you don't necessarily move through them in order. They are numbness, searching and pining, depression, and recovery.

Other models of loss describe denial, anger, bargaining, depression, and acceptance. The reality is you might have all or none of these and experience a range of emotions in the space of a day. You might feel like you will never accept it or recover, but you learn to live with the scar. Everyone's experience of loss is unique, and there is no right way to grieve.

Analogies can help us understand what loss can feel like, such as the ball in the box. Imagine a box with a ball in it,[41] and a pain button on the inside. In the beginning – after a loss – the ball is

---

[40] *Bereavement: Studies of Grief in Adult Life.* Dr Colin Murray Parkes (2013)
[41] Lauren Herschel @LaurenHerschel

huge, taking up most of the box. You can't move without the ball hitting the pain button over and over. You cannot control it, and it can feel relentless. Over time, the ball gets smaller, so it hits the pain button less, but it still hurts as much when it does. You start to be able to function day to day, although the ball can randomly hit the pain button for no apparent reason. Some days, the ball might feel bigger – such as anniversaries, holidays, birthdays, or when you see reminders. Being able to describe how big the ball feels can be a helpful way to put grief into words.

This description of grief can also be helpful: "Grief, I have learned, is just love. It is all the love you want to give but cannot. All that unspent love gathers in the corners of your eyes, the lump in your throat, and in the hollow part of your chest. Grief is just love with no place to go."[42]

Sarah Stevenson lost her parents, Roy and Diana, within three months of each other to cancer when she was 28 years old. She describes her experience of loss. "It is a physical pain in your chest and stomach, a ball of pain where you can't breathe. I would go to the physio and say I was in pain, but there wasn't anything physically wrong; it was the stress showing up in my body.

"Whilst my parents were undergoing treatment, I had an extra gear when training as I thought 'if they can deal with their pain, I can push harder'. When they died, this disappeared and I was in survival mode. I was angry a lot; why had this happened to them? They are good people. I was angry at people who got frustrated over trivial things in life and were moaning when nothing bad had happened to them.

"Grief can change you as a person, so I have also grieved for the person I was before. I lost my source of unconditional love, and I didn't feel safe; the people who would be there for me – no matter what – had gone. Feeling unsafe meant I wanted to control everything and know every detail of what was going to happen. I had this tendency before, but grief exaggerated it tenfold. This stopped me enjoying life, so eventually, I had to get tough with myself and start living again.

---

[42] Jamie Anderson, author of Dr Who.

"I can still have a bad day and get upset, but it doesn't stop me. People told me time would help, which I didn't want to hear, but it is true. You must go through the pain; no one can take that away. I found talking to others and understanding that my experiences were understandable helpful. You notice when you have lost someone that people don't know what to say, so can ignore you. This is hard and feels so awkward. It would be great if people could be brave and say, 'I'm sorry, I don't know what to say, but I don't want to ignore you' or give you a hug.

"I wish my parents were still here, but losing them has given me perspective on life, and I have passed on my parents' values to my kids. It makes me think about what people would say about you when you die, so I want to live a life I am proud of."

It can be hard to be appreciative of the time you had with the person you have lost if it is gone too soon. "It is better to have loved and lost than never to have loved at all"[43] reminds us to try to appreciate this. People can find solace by keeping their memories alive and talking about them. Others find writing a letter to the person they have lost helpful. The Good Grief Trust provides information, advice, and stories that can be reassuring, as well as pop-up cafes to meet others in similar situations.[44]

It is important not to make assumptions about the impact of a loss on someone else. We never know the depth of connection they had. Rachelle Booth described how – when she lost her grandfather – people expected her to get over it quickly and didn't realise the strength of their bond. "I spoke to him every day, so it was a massive loss. It is hard to care about anything. It impacted on my ability to train. I learnt to cope with it in healthier ways, but it took time."

The ending of a relationship (romantic or otherwise) often results in intense feelings of grief that we need to give ourselves time to experience. There is no set timescale that this should happen in. It can impact on our feelings of self-worth if the ending was painful and difficult, so support from others to reinforce our worth helps.

---

[43] Quote from the poem by Alfred Lord Tennyson.

[44] www.the goodgrieftrust.org

Summary

- Relationships are the best and worst things for our mental health, so it is worth investing time in developing good relationships and avoiding unhealthy ones
- How we act in relationships is shaped by interactions with parents/caregivers and early life experiences, and as we grow, we establish patterns of interacting that can be helpful (or unhelpful) in living the life we want. Being aware of them is the first step to developing alternatives
- Being able to recognise and manage our emotions has a positive impact on mental health
- It is important to recognise if a relationship is good or unhealthy, whilst understanding how these fluctuate on a spectrum
- There are many ways to improve your relationships, but the best way is to fully listen, understand, and empathise
- A good athlete-coach relationship is important for influencing sporting outcomes and mental health. Good relationships often have commitment, closeness, and collaboration
- Developing the skills of having difficult conversations and receiving feedback will benefit you in sport and in life
- Loss is a sad reality of life and is something we should understand and talk about

Chapter 5: Managing stress, fear, and anxiety

- What are stress, fear, and anxiety?
- How do you recognise and manage them, so they don't derail your performances and impact on your mental health?

Stress, fear, and anxiety are terms that are often used interchangeably, and which can have similar impacts on your body, but there are differences that are worth understanding. Figuring out which ones you are experiencing will help you deal with them more effectively. These are *vital* skills if you want to thrive in sport and life.

Stress

This is when there is a *demand* that causes you to *get ready for action*. Energy is directed to parts of the body such as the heart, lungs, and muscles, with less going to other areas like the digestive system. Your awareness also narrows and alertness levels increase.

Stressors can be physical or psychological. They might include: a cold room where your body shivers to keep warm, lifting heavy weights, a difficult conversation (or imagining having one), or lots of activities to fit into a day. Once the stressor has gone, your body should return to a calm state. Stress – in the right amount with the right recovery – is good for us. You can have stress with or without fear and anxiety.

Fear

This is an emotion that shares many of the physiological responses with stress and anxiety, such as increased heart rate and breathing. There is a *perception* of immediate threat in the moment or a memory of a past threat. Your brain wants to keep you safe and avoid negative consequences, so you get a fight, flight, or freeze response.

To keep safe, I will attack, run away, or do nothing/tune out from what is going on (disassociation). An example of fear might see you on a start line and seeing the task ahead of you as threatening, as you don't feel prepared. You might have had an injury and the fear of it happening again means you are scared to push yourself.

Anxiety

Anxiety is thinking about the future and imagining or predicting threat. This consists of thoughts and physiological responses such as sweaty palms, high heart rate, quickened breathing, or tension in your muscles and jaw. You might imagine something going wrong when you next compete and have thoughts such as 'What if I am not fit enough? What if I mess up(?)... I could get injured.'

Stress, fear, and anxiety are understandable experiences, given how our minds work as they try to keep us safe. Stress, fear, and anxiety can lead to trouble sleeping, concentrating, enjoying life, and performing how you want to. They can impact on your mood and how you interact with others; you might become more irritable, angrier, or quieter than usual. If you have high levels of demands in your life – that are not well-managed – they can increase the likelihood of injury due to inattention, distraction, increased muscle tension, and impaired coordination. So, managing stress is important (for the sake of you, your relationships, and your performance)! As a way of coping, we might use strategies such as avoidance or numbing that help in the short term but not in the long term.

What influences whether you experience stress, fear, or anxiety?

You might have noticed that your ability to deal with challenges in life can vary over time. Below are some examples of factors that play a part:

- Your personality
- Past life experiences
- How others around you respond to challenges
- The number of challenges you are currently facing
- How tired you are

- Your comfort or familiarity with the situation
- Your menstrual cycle, in females
- Your support networks

Whilst you can only influence some of these factors, it can be useful to acknowledge them to help you understand why you feel the way you do. We saw in Chapter 4 how important it is to develop good relationships and what to do if you experience fear and anxiety due to relationship issues. Having good relationships and support to tackle fears and worries is helpful.

Stress (cont.)

Let's delve a bit deeper into stress. People often say, 'I feel so stressed; my stress levels are sky-high,' and stress can get a bad press when, in fact, it shouldn't.

The complete absence of stress is not good for us.

Imagine sitting on a beach all day, every day, with nothing to do. The idea might sound great, but the novelty soon wears off and you would need some stimulation and challenge. Getting the amount of stress right for you, and having time to recover, is crucial. It works like a see-saw. The stressor activates the body, so it is ready for action, tipping the see-saw to one side and releasing adrenaline and cortisol (the sympathetic nervous system is activated). After the stress has gone, the see-saw tips back the other way to the calming system (the parasympathetic nervous system).

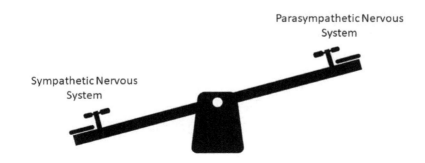

Short-term stress has positive impacts and can help immune function, alertness, and focus. If you spend too long on the 'ready for action' side with high levels of adrenaline in your body, though, it can have negative impacts such as weakening your immune system and affecting your sleep. All the demands in your life combine and contribute to the level of stress on your body and brain, so – as well as training – you could have work, study, exams, life admin, and difficult relationships to contend with.

Ideas for managing stress

We will look at three strategies:

1. Remove or reduce the source of stress
2. Reinterpret the source of stress
3. Recover from demands

Remove or reduce

Sometimes, it is possible to remove or reduce sources of stress; for example, if you have got a week of exams or lots of meetings, you might reduce the number of training sessions you do or say no to an event you have been invited to. If a relationship is difficult, you might consider ways to improve it. This is called *problem-focused coping*. You could:

- Plan and pre-empt harder weeks of training and check other commitments to avoid overload. Have a planner that shows all activities
- Prioritise what is most important each week, based on the bigger picture (this will help you make good decisions). You can create a rating system that helps you determine what the important things are, which stops things that seem urgent (but are not) taking over your day
- Make life easier by setting reminders and finding the most efficient way to do things. Having a packing list for trips will help save time and energy, for example
- Ask for help if you need it

Not everyone finds planning easy. If a lack of planning and organising is making it hard to manage the demands placed on you, then find a planning process that works for you. This might be sitting down on Sunday night and mapping out the week ahead.

Planning frees up mental energy to do more of the things you enjoy.

In the moment stress – If you feel like there are demands on you, and you want to feel calmer in that moment, then this breathing exercise is the quickest way to achieve that. Telling yourself (or someone else telling you) to just calm down usually doesn't work!

This breathing exercise is called the *physiological sigh*[45] and involves taking two inhales through your nose, followed by a long, vigorous exhale. The exhale needs to be longer than the inhales. Repeat this several times. The breathing process activates the calming parasympathetic system and slows down breathing and heart rate. Try taking your pulse before and after you do this to see the impact. Looking wide at the horizon or taking in the whole room (rather than having tunnel vision) also helps bring a sense of calm.

Building stress tolerance – As mentioned, small doses of stress are good for us. Choosing to put yourself into a situation where demands are placed on you and learning to tolerate them helps build your ability to cope. It is the same principle you use for building your physical strength. One way to do this is through cold exposure, such as ice baths or cold showers, with water below 15 degrees Celsius. You can learn to breathe and relax your mind whilst your body is placed under stress.

Make sure you only access cold water when it is safe, and you are not putting yourself or others at risk. People report feeling wonderful afterwards. Another way to build tolerance is to gradually expose yourself to demands in training that are as close as possible to those you will face in competition.

Reinterpret

The meaning you make of something has a powerful influence on your thoughts, feelings, and behaviours. The view that stress is all bad is not accurate or helpful. A study[46] following people over an 18-year period found those who believed stress was good for them

---

[45] https://youtu.be/PZ-GvIOhcf8 Dr Andrew Huberman.

[46] Keller, A. *et al.* (2012) Does the perception that stress affects health matter? The Association with Health and Mortality. *Health Psychology.*

were healthier, lived longer, and had better regulation of adrenaline and cortisol. This mindset reduced the 'stress about stress' and allowed people to make better decisions.

Think of times when the demands of a situation helped you to focus or perform. Be aware of how often you use the word 'stressed' or say 'this situation is a nightmare' when it isn't that bad. Language is powerful, so choose your words wisely!

Adrenaline not nerves – When a demand is placed on you, adrenaline is released to get you ready for action. How you interpret this adrenaline release is important – if you see it as a sign that your body is ready, and will benefit from it, this is much more helpful than seeing it as a sign of nerves and something to be worried about.

Some people find adrenaline in their body more unpleasant than others as it can make you feel sick, have sweaty palms, and a dry mouth, but you can learn to understand these physiological aspects and see them as a positive sign. Say to yourself, 'I am ready' instead of 'I feel nervous.'

- Are there any aspects of your life that you currently perceive as difficult that you could see another way? If you can reinterpret them as a challenge, or even find some enjoyment in them, they will place fewer demands on you mentally. Imagine you are in an airport security queue and it is taking longer than expected. You can either see this as frustrating and annoying, or accept it and be glad that you are going on a trip
- Gaining perspective and having realistic expectations can help reduce how difficult something seems. If things go smoothly, it is a bonus… but be ready if they don't. In the grand scheme of life, how difficult is this situation to deal with?
- Tolerating frustration in life has a positive influence on mental health. Being able to recognise how you are feeling, pausing, and then deciding if you want to go with that feeling or see things another way is a vital skill for managing stress. Rather than thinking, 'Why has this happened to me?' think, 'How can I deal with this?'

> *Activity*
>
> Write down the current demands on your mind and body.
>
> Are there any ways you could remove or reduce any demands?
>
> Is there anything you see as difficult that could be reinterpreted?

Recovery

We need to ensure we tip the see-saw back and turn off the stress response. If you don't recover, it gets harder to maintain energy, and manage your emotions and focus. If your sleep is not how you want it to be, this could be a sign you are not managing demands as well as you could. Chapter 6 covers ways that we can switch off and recover from demanding occasions.

Fear

Do you find things scary or threatening in the moment, or do you have a memory of a past threat?

Fear is subjective. We can fear different things depending on what we perceive as threatening. This could be a threat to your physical body (such as getting injured), or a psychological threat (such as how you see yourself, how others see you, or doubting your ability).

The fear response can be a good thing as it keeps us alive and stops us from making poor decisions; it also makes sense from a survival point of view to detect threat readily. When we see something as threatening that need not be, or it stops us living life how we want to, then we need to learn how to manage it.

Just one difficult experience is enough to develop a fear response, unlike other types of learning, which can take much longer. Being in difficult and scary situations while you are growing up means your threat detection could be easily triggered, as your mind learnt the world is not a safe place. Imagine a smoke detector that goes off when you slightly burn the toast.

Here is an example of how fear can develop, based on a person's beliefs.

Alex was competing at an event that was going to be used for team selection. This event was important to him, and training had gone well, so he had high expectations. The whole family were watching and supporting. When Alex arrived at the venue, he felt sick, and his heart rate was high, which felt unpleasant, and he saw these as signs something bad was going to happen. Alex wanted to get the event over with.

Alex made a mistake early on and found it hard to regain focus, so didn't perform as well as he usually did in training. Alex saw his family's faces and decided they looked upset as they had travelled a long way to watch him. Alex didn't get selected and felt awful about himself. Whilst competing in his next event, Alex felt dread and fear.

Ideas for managing fear

Managing an experience from the past that felt threatening:

- *Tell the story* of the threatening experience, describing how you *felt* rather than just the facts. This might give you similar physiological responses to those you had at the time, so you could feel uncomfortable. What was the worst thing about the story, and what it means about you? The story needs to be repeated on several occasions until it becomes boring, and the responses reduce or go away. If the experience was extremely difficult or distressing, you might need professional support to do this
- *What did you see as threatening in that situation?* What beliefs about yourself or others underpin your fear? Writing them down enables you to explore them and see how accurate and helpful these beliefs are, and helps you formulate new beliefs
- *Create a new story.* You need to replace the story with a new one with an updated meaning. For Alex, the original meaning was, "I am useless, and I let everyone down; I shouldn't have made a mistake, and I can't cope if it happens again." Change the meaning by creating a new story that allows you to be in the same situation in the future with a different perspective. For athletes like Alex, this could be, "The selection event was important to me;

I showed courage by competing. Mistakes will happen; this experience has shown me I can work on improving how I manage my mind and interpret the adrenaline in my body. My mind was just trying to keep me safe, but it wasn't needed." You can then practise the ideas in the competition section later in this chapter and reinforce new beliefs

- *Then v now.*[47] You can remind yourself about what is different now compared to the time you perceived the threat. It could be that you have more experience, you have learnt tools to manage your mind, you have generated new meaning from the experience, or you have talked to those important to you and got their support and advice
- *Rewards.* When we perceive a threat, negative consequences sit at the front of our minds. Before you get into the situation, reinforce the rewards and reasons as to why you are doing it. Often, you start competing because you enjoy your sport, so try to reconnect to this. Rewards could be the satisfaction of completing the challenge or pushing yourself out of your comfort zone. Tell yourself you have chosen to be here. The swimmer Adam Peaty[48] has said, "Pressure doesn't exist. It is an artificial thing that's a cloud that some people carry and some shove away. I enjoy racing because I want to do it. No one is forcing me. What is the worst that could happen? I lose a race?"
- *Facts.* Knowing the facts about a situation can help reduce fear. If you fear flying, for example, an experienced pilot explaining why turbulence happens, that the plane can handle it, and that flying is the safest form of transport could help
- *Faith.* Having a religious faith can help people manage their fears

---

[47] *Be Extraordinary: 7 Key Skills to Transform Your Life from Ordinary to Extraordinary.* Dr Jennifer Wild (2020)

[48] @adam_peaty

- *Don't avoid the situation.* To try to keep you safe, your mind might tell you to avoid what you see as threatening. This just reinforces that there is something to be feared and the longer you leave it, the harder it gets. Your mind needs to experience being in the situation to realise that nothing bad happens. You might need to do this gradually; for example, competing at a smaller or lower-level event. *You can feel fear and still take action despite it*

In the moment fear

It is best to manage perceptions of threats before you get into the situation, but sometimes you will still experience in the moment fear.

- You can manage physiological aspects such as high heart rate and quickened breathing using the physiological sigh (from the stress section above) to help induce calm (double inhale through your nose, long vigorous exhale), or finger trace breathing (breathe in through your nose as you trace up your thumb with your other hand, breathe out as you trace down. Repeat with each finger)
- Use distractions such as music, singing, talking to someone, or playing a game
- Ground yourself in the present moment by sitting on the floor, describing what you can see, hear, touch, naming as many blue/red/yellow objects as possible
- Focus on a plan and aspects in your control (have these ready beforehand)
- Get support from those around you, preferably those who are calm and reassuring

Panic attacks

A panic attack is a sudden intense feeling of fear that can feel scary and out of control, lasting between 5 and 20 minutes. Some people describe it as feeling like they are having a heart attack, are going to faint, or even die. You get physiological sensations such as tingling in your hands and feet, dizziness, sweating, high heart rate, ringing in your ears, difficulty breathing, feeling sick or shaking.

The fear of having an attack and how that feels, as well as what others might think, can be distressing, especially as you don't know when they will happen. Some people only have one or two in their life; for others, it is more often. It is important to see a doctor to rule out any underlying medical issues.

It is difficult to pinpoint a single cause of panic attacks as they can vary from person to person. Factors could include past or current life experiences and worries. Talking to a professional and learning to manage anxiety daily is beneficial. Knowing that although they feel difficult, they are not dangerous, and they will pass can be reassuring. Some people repeat a phrase such as 'This will pass' during an attack. Having a plan ready if an attack happens can help reduce the anticipatory fear. Focusing on your breathing will help, using diaphragmatic/belly breathing[49] or the physiological sigh. Practise this when you are feeling calm, as it will make it easier to use during an attack. Grounding techniques such as sitting on the floor, touching or squeezing an object, and focusing on your surroundings also help. You might want to tell people about the possibility of having an attack, so they know how to support you in the moment.

Anxiety

Do you think about the future and imagine or predict threat, or not being able to cope?

Life is unpredictable, and we don't live forever, so it is not surprising that we often imagine what might happen in the future. Vivid imagination allows humans to be creative and achieve amazing feats, but we can also use it to picture the worst.

How often do you think about the future and picture it going well versus badly? How often do you imagine what someone else is thinking about you? If you don't like heights, you could imagine

---

[49] Place one hand on the top of your chest and the other below your rib cage. When you breathe in slowly and deeply, you will feel your diaphragm moving. As you breathe in slowly, you want to feel your belly move out against your hand. The hand on your chest should not move.

being on a high bridge and get the same thoughts and physiological sensations as if you were standing on it.

From a survival perspective, it makes sense to anticipate what could go wrong, so you are not caught off guard. Anxiety can feel vague and tough to pin down to a specific thing, which can make it seem harder to deal with. It can make small tasks seem daunting and overwhelming and leave you feeling exhausted.

'What if' is a favourite phrase when someone is feeling anxious, and we tend to get stuck wondering and worrying. An athlete told me how their coach would encourage them to focus on the now and cross the bridge when they came to it rather than worrying about what might happen. They said how – in their mind – they had already fallen off the bridge into the water and been eaten by a shark.

There can be an underlying belief that worrying will stop bad things happening, thus serving a purpose, when logically we know this is not true.

Due to their personalities, some people are more comfortable with uncertainty or feel more optimistic about the future than others, which will impact on how anxious they feel. When you are tired, or have lots of demands in your life, you might feel more anxious. Our brains are constantly getting inputs from the outside world and internally from our own bodies. When we feel anxious, our focus is usually internal, on our thoughts and bodily sensations. Noticing these sensations can reinforce the view that we are anxious – 'My heart is racing, so I must be anxious.'

Ideas for managing anxiety

- You can *manage physiological aspects,* such as high heart rate and quickened breathing, using the physiological sigh from the stress section above to help induce calm (double inhale through your nose, long vigorous exhale). Practise muscle relaxation techniques where you learn to contract and relax each part of your body
- Write down what you are *worried might happen,* being as specific as you can be. If you can't pin it down to a specific thing, it is likely to be a worry that you won't be able to cope. Write down the resources you have within yourself

and support from those around you that will help you cope. Remind yourself of the difficult things you have coped with in the past. This will help you gain perspective

- *What if statements.* Instead of saying 'What if I lose?', write it down as a concrete statement such as 'I don't want to lose as my coach will think I am not improving.' With each statement, ask yourself – is it true? How do I know? What do I want to happen, and what can I control or influence that gives it the best chance of happening?
- *What if planning.* You can't predict every scenario, but you can work out the most likely ones, or ones you are most anxious about. Have a plan ready for how you would deal with each one. The swimmer Michael Phelps managed to win gold at the Beijing Olympic Games despite his goggles filling with water and having no visibility for the last 50 meters of the race. He would practice swimming without goggles in training, so he was ready if this happened. Some athletes find it helpful to picture the worst-case scenario and reassure themselves that they would cope, and it isn't life and death
- *What if it goes well?* When you notice yourself picturing something going badly, see if you can create an alternative image where it goes well. What are you doing that helps it to go well? This will remind you what you need to focus on
- *Practise shifting your focus from internal to external.* An internal focus would be noticing your heart rate, how fast you are breathing, how full your stomach is, the feeling of clothes against your skin, and your thoughts. An external focus would be focusing on something in your environment and noticing as many details as you can. The more you practice this, the better you will get at being able to shift this focus when you want to, and it will help you get out of your own head
- *Acceptance.* This is used in therapies such as Acceptance Commitment Therapy. You notice and accept the thoughts you are having rather than fighting them. You create distance between you and your thoughts as a reminder that you are not your thoughts. Just because you

have a thought that something might go wrong does not mean it will, and you don't have to engage with it
- *Problem-solving process.* If you have a process that you can apply in any situation, this can be reassuring. Talking to someone else often helps this process. An example is the 5-step process (1. Define the problem. 2. Gather information. 3. Generate possible solutions. 4. Evaluate ideas and choose one. 5. Review how it is going.)
- *Have a plan for the day.* This can help you to focus on aspects within your control. If it feels hard to get started on a task, break it down into smaller parts or tell yourself you will do it for a few minutes, then stop. This helps to overcome the feeling of it being a huge task
- *Flow.* If you do an activity that you enjoy and can get engrossed in, it will help you be in the moment rather than thinking about the future
- Avoid *alcohol* or *stimulants* such as caffeine

Checklist

Use the table below to capture what helps you. You can create this with those who support you or share it with them.

Strategies	How will I put this into practice
Breathing exercises	
Writing down worries and reassuring answers	
What if planning	
What if it goes well	
Shifting my focus from internal to external	
Notice and accept my thoughts are not facts	

Strategies	How will I put this into practice
Have a problem-solving process	
Have a plan for the day	

Shame and embarrassment

At the root of stress, fear, and anxiety often lies feelings of embarrassment and shame. Many athletes say they feel like this after a performance they are not happy with. We experience shame if we don't feel good enough and don't feel worthy as a person.[50] People often describe an underlying feeling that they have done something wrong or are living under the gaze of a critic.

If self-worth is linked to outcomes, then there is a high likelihood of feeling shame and embarrassment. We often set ourselves a standard that we want to achieve, or think others *expect* us to achieve, then feel bad if we don't meet it. Jade Jones described feeling embarrassed after losing in Tokyo and feeling anxious in the run-up, imagining what people would think about her if she didn't win. After Tokyo, she realised how supportive everyone was, and her fears were not realised. People valued her for putting herself in the fight for a third gold medal.

Shame is based on our view of what others think about us on aspects such as how good we are at sport, our appearance, health, identity, qualifications, etc. Feelings of shame have been linked to poor mental health, as we just don't feel good about ourselves.

Consider how shame shows up in your body and how it feels. We often want to shrink down and avoid people or eye contact.

We all feel fear and anxiety, but the need to seem strong can stop us talking about them. Keeping things to yourself and avoiding them only fuels the fire. Being vulnerable and sharing that you feel fear, anxiety, and shame with someone who will empathise and

---

[50] https://www.ted.com/talks/brene_brown_the_power_of_vulnerability?language=en

not judge can help. It will help you feel less alone, understand what your fears and worries are, and work out strategies that can help. It can feel emotionally risky to do this, so make sure it is someone you trust.

As we saw in Chapter 3, basing self-worth on more than just outcomes in sport helps to reduce fear and anxiety. By being vulnerable and sharing how you feel when you don't perform how you want to, you can take steps to manage it and reduce feelings of embarrassment.

In the chapter on relationships, we saw that it is helpful to understand and care what certain people in our lives think about us. If you want a good quality relationship, then knowing how we feel about each other matters. In a good relationship, the other person will value you not just on the outcomes you get in sport. They might be disappointed *for you* but not with you. The golfer Scottie Scheffler said, "My identity isn't a golf score. Like Meredith (my wife) told me this morning, if you win this golf tournament, if you lose by ten shots, if you never win another golf tournament again, I'm still going to love you; you are still the same person."

Sadly, some people might show their own disappointment or annoyance at how you performed. This might be a temporary reaction when – deep down – they know you did your best and didn't deliberately go out to underperform. If this is how they feel, even when they have calmed down, you need to protect yourself from the impacts of their behaviour. You might be able to let them know how this makes you feel, and how it leads to more fear and anxiety the next time you compete, or you might need to limit or cut contact. The likelihood is they judge themselves by outcomes as well.

Problems arise when we care what *everyone* thinks. Firstly, there is no way of knowing or influencing this, and it is unrealistic for the whole world to think you are great. Most people are so caught up in their own lives that they don't give you much thought, or not for very long. The key is to work out which relationships are important to you and accept you can't control what people outside of this group think.

Compassion

If you feel shame, you are likely to be critical of yourself, and believe others are critical of you. Compassion can be the antidote.

When you think of compassion, what does it mean to you?

Compassion is *not* letting yourself off the hook, being weak, giving yourself pity or accepting underperformance. To be compassionate to yourself, or someone else, means being able to understand and engage with suffering/distress and *doing something about it rather than avoiding it.*[51]

It is a motivation to notice and improve things. If you are feeling anxious, being compassionate to yourself would mean acknowledging how you feel and taking action to manage it. This is not always easy, and we might need others to help.

It takes courage to show compassion. Compassion is acknowledging that everyone suffers and feels pain; we are not alone in our experiences. This helps us to feel able to share how we feel with others rather than isolating ourselves. It is not 'just me' who feels like this; life goes wrong for everyone at some point. The opposite of compassion is avoiding or dismissing feelings, judging, and criticising.

Compassion can flow in three ways:

1. Self to others
2. Others to self
3. Self to self

Many people find it easier to be compassionate to others and find it hard to receive or show it to themselves. Often, we berate ourselves for feeling shame, anxiety, or fear which only makes it worse. 'I am such an idiot; what is wrong with me? Why can't I just do this? I shouldn't be feeling like this.'

What do you say to yourself when you are being self-critical? This self-punishment and judgement often goes unnoticed as it becomes a habit, but it can cause us pain. It can take practice to

---

[51] https://self-compassion.org/ Kristin Neff

develop self-compassion, especially if you have not experienced it from others in your life.

Those who develop a compassionate inner voice have been found to learn more quickly than those who are self-critical. They have lower levels of anxiety and are better able to tackle difficulties in life.

Compassion can be direct and forceful if needed. If a child is walking towards a main road, you would grab them in an urgent and forceful way. In other words, a soft approach is not always what is needed, but it should always be non-judgemental and with the aim of relieving distress. Imagine someone you care about sitting in front of you, and you wanted to tell them something. Picture yourself saying it in three different tones – neutral, critical/mocking, and warm and caring. How did each one feel? What tone does your inner voice have? Is it critical or warm? You can create an image for your critical voice. What does it look and sound like?

It can help to develop an image of a compassionate person and think how they would be with you. This can be a real person or an imaginary one. Ideally, they would have qualities such as:

- Accepting how you are feeling without judgement
- Able to handle your distress
- Help you to find ways to manage it
- Are wise
- Challenging in a supportive way

When you are struggling, you could imagine what this person would say or do. You can then start to develop a compassionate part in yourself, using phrases they would use. You can imagine the compassionate part talking to the critical part. The critical part might be trying to protect you and keep you safe, but it does it in an unhelpful way. The internal conversation might look like this:

Critical: What is wrong with you? Why did you make that mistake? You looked stupid.

Compassionate: I know you are trying to protect me and stop me from being rejected. It feels painful when we make a mistake. I want to avoid mistakes as well. I didn't go out to mess up; I lost focus when we were losing. I am going to practise refocusing during training.

Some view their inner critic as the fuel that drives them, and worry that if they lose this, they won't try as hard. If you develop and listen to the compassionate inner voice, you can be driven by challenge and opportunity rather than threat, which is usually more enjoyable and results in better outcomes.

> *Activity*
>
> Have you felt shame or embarrassment, and how did it feel in your body?
>
> How can you develop your compassionate inner voice? What would it say?

Sources of stress, fear, and anxiety

In sport, and in life, it is inevitable that challenges and adversity will come our way. There are aspects of the sporting environment that are inherent, such as rankings, selection, getting feedback, injuries, and illness, so we need to learn how to manage them the best we can.

We will discuss the following:

- Injuries and illness
- Competition
- Personal life
- Transitions

Other sources of stress include relationships and the environment you are in. These have been covered in Chapters 2 and 4.

Injuries and illness

Understandably, an injury or illness can be difficult to manage mentally, with injured athletes reporting more anxiety than noninjured athletes. 80% of the time, athletes coming for treatment to an injury also discuss psychological issues related to the injury.[52]

Below are common difficulties and concerns expressed by injured athletes:

- Everyone else is getting better
- I won't come back at the level I was at before
- I miss the structure and rewards I get from training and competing
- I feel isolated
- Is this the right treatment plan?
- What if it happens again?

This can lead to returning too soon, doing too much, or feeling unmotivated to do the rehabilitation needed to recover.

Lauren Williams, a taekwondo fighter, has had more than her fair share of injuries. "The hardest thing about being injured is being out of training; I worry about the training I am missing and how I am going to catch up. The frustration of wanting to train, wanting to adapt sessions to stay involved but not being able to, is challenging, especially when it is all you know and enjoy. Watching the team carry on training while you are sat on the sidelines playing the waiting game is hard."

Ideas for managing injuries

Social support – It is easy to become isolated if you can't train with other people. Form a group with other injured athletes or arrange to meet up with friends and teammates. Support from others when we are facing challenges helps us to cope more effectively. You might not feel like being sociable, but isolation is likely to give you more time to dwell.

Reformulate your plan and understand the milestones – The first step is to accept you are injured and cannot do what you normally would. You need to let go of your previous plans and formulate a new one. If you understand your injury and your rehabilitation plan, you are more likely to be able to contribute and commit to a new

---

[52] Wolanin, A., Gross, M., and Hon, E. (2015) Depression in Athletes. *Current Sports Medicine Reports.*

plan. It will help you understand which activities will help and hinder your recovery.

Athletes often want exact dates of when they can return or progress to the next stage, whereas they are likely to be given milestones. This is because everyone's body responds differently, and medical professionals will want to ensure progress has been made before moving to the next level. If you are working with professionals who understand sport, they will want you to return as quickly as possible. You can tick off the milestones as you reach them and remind yourself how – if you follow the plan – you will reach each one more quickly. If you rush, you will take one step forward and two back.

Lauren said she has learnt that injuries heal with time and should be respected. "If I could go back to 15-year-old Lauren, when injuries first started occurring, I would say accept an injury earlier on; it has happened, and it is not going to change. Focus on what I can do now and find alternative ways to train and stay engaged given what I can do."

Develop your skills – It is possible to continue to develop knowledge and skills relevant to your sport while you are injured. This could be watching videos, discussing tactics, and visualising yourself performing (see the Appendix for visualisation tips). Lauren describes how she does this. "I stay tactically engaged, watching fights, watching opponents, and keeping my competition mind focused. It really does help because, when I get back to fitness and my injuries allow me to start competitive training again, I only have to wait for my fitness to catch up. I have done the work in my head during the time I have been out, so I haven't missed as much as I think."

Successful comeback stories – No one has perfect preparation, always free from injury and illness. Listening to stories of athletes who have overcome injuries can reassure you it can be done. The golfer Tiger Woods has struggled with injuries for most of his career. He ruptured an ACL in 2007, his Achilles tendon in 2008, then had back injuries from 2014 onwards. Following back surgery, he went on to win the Masters in 2019. NFL player Tom Brady was on the injury report 186 times in his 17-year career, including a torn ACL and MCL in his knee. I have witnessed numerous athletes come back from injury and achieve more than they did before!

Values – If you have worked out what is important to you in life, you can find activities that match them – that you can do while injured. If challenge was one of your values, you could find activities that provide this, such as learning a new language. Having other interests and identities helps when you are injured.

Optimism – Higher levels of optimism are associated with improved recovery from injury. You can see this as an opportunity to strengthen your body during your rehabilitation and work on your mental skills. If you see injury as a disaster and difficult to cope with, the levels of adrenaline and cortisol in your system will be higher for longer. This will impact on your immune system and slow down healing times. Feeling anxious impacts on how we perceive pain, so it is important to acknowledge and manage your worries.

The runner Pippa Woolven described how she made framing her injury as a positive into a game. "I tore my calf, and it would be easy to fall into the trap of feeling down and frustrated about it. Instead, I decided to see if I could enjoy the rehab process and see bike sessions as a new challenge. It is easy to lose perspective, so you need to remind yourself you will recover and each day you are getting closer to returning."

People living with chronic pain have the difficult task of learning how to manage this day to day.[53]

Focus on the process when you return – It is understandable that your mind will want to protect you and make sure you don't get injured again. This can lead to hesitation and fear. You can get reassurance from medical professionals that you have recovered enough to train, but then you need to manage your mind. Remind yourself that when you hesitate and overthink, you are more likely to get injured. The ideas for managing fear in the section above will help. Focus on what you can control, so you know you are doing the best you can to avoid injury.

---

[53] *Master Your Chronic Pain: A Practical Guide.* Dr Nicola Sherlock (2021)

Competition

- Confidence
- Frustrations
- Dealing with disappointment

When you compete, how do you feel? Is it excitement, nerves, fear, anxiety, or a mix of feelings? One factor given by many athletes that influences their feelings at a competition is their confidence levels.

Confidence

What does confidence mean to you? 'I don't feel confident today' or 'my confidence is high after that session.' Confidence can be described as trusting your ability to meet the demands of a situation.

Imagine walking along a narrow plank of wood placed on the floor. You wouldn't need to think about it; you just do it. Now the plank is raised to the height of a house. How do you feel about walking along it? The task is the same, but there is a consequence if you make a mistake. This is the same in a sporting context. There is the ability to carry out the physical, technical, and tactical parts of your sport, plus the ability to manage your mind, to allow you to perform at your best when there is a consequence. You need to have a plan for both parts.

Ability to carry out the physical, technical, and tactical parts of your sport

Evidence – It is important to understand your strengths and have evidence to remind you of them on competition day. It is easy to lose sight of them and doubt your ability. When you practise something, it eventually becomes automatic, meaning you don't need to give it much conscious thought. Trusting that your strengths are automatic is vital for confidence.

Evidence could include videos of you performing skills or tactics, a reminder of your preparation, or a list of your strengths. Reassurance about your strengths from someone you trust can also be helpful. Accept where your skills and fitness are on the day of competition, so you can make the best of them.

Ability to manage your mind when there is a consequence

Choose the mindset you want on competition day – Write down how you want to be. This might include: focused, enjoying it, seeing it as a challenge. You can get ideas from the 'approaches to sport' section in Chapter 2.

Face consequences and fears – Rather than ignoring thoughts about consequences, you need to face and address them. They don't go away if you ignore them. Which consequences are causing you distress? What could interfere with the mindset you want to have? Write them down and examine each one. Can you change the meaning you give to the consequence? Can you find an answer that reassures you? Consequences are usually out of our control, so accept that and shift the focus to things you can control, which leads us to the point below.

Plan/process – Having a plan for competition day and a process to focus on while competing enables you to focus on what is in your control. No matter how big the consequence is, this is what will give you the best chance of performing at your best. You want to allow the automatic part of your mind to be activated, as it would when you are training and enjoying yourself (when something is well practised, it becomes automatic and quick). Athletes can get to an event and think they need to try harder, so end up overthinking.

To see the impact of this, pick an activity that is automatic – such as driving a car – and think about everything you are doing. It can feel strange and clunky, and decisions are slower. It is common that fear and anxiety take over, which also stops the automatic part of your mind from working effectively.

Reflect on your best performances in training or competition and write down what you were thinking about or focusing on. It is likely that there wasn't a whole lot of conscious thinking going on, just a few focus points or reminders.

Dr Geir Jordet is a professor at the Norwegian School of Sport Sciences. He spent five years analysing every penalty shootout since 1976 at the World Cup and Euro finals and interviewed a number of players. He found that if players took less or more time than usual to take a penalty kick, they were more likely to miss. This is because they are consciously thinking about an automatic action. Marcus Rashford, by way of example, waited 11 seconds during the Euro 2020 shootout before missing.

Write down your process or focus points that help you get into the automatic mode when you compete. Visualising how you want to compete can also help you get into this mode (see Appendix).

"The result today is important to me; I want to perform at my best. I can't control what the outcome is, or what others will do, so I am going to focus on my process. This will give me the best chance. If I make a mistake, I will accept it and refocus back on my plan." Golfer Annika Sorenstam would focus on the 'now' shot, rather than dwelling on the past shot or mistake.

Choice – No one is making you compete (I hope). When you get to an event and feel fear and anxiety, it can help to remind yourself that you have chosen to be here. You want this challenge.

Focus on rewards – For some athletes, it helps them if they focus on the rewards they will get from competing, and the thought of the outcome drives them to commit. They enjoy the element of competition and consequence and use it to their advantage.

Doing your best – If you focus on doing your best in the situation you are in, with the preparation you have had, there is nothing else you can do. We often look back in hindsight and think, 'I could have done that better' but – at the time – that was the best you had. It can help to make a list of all the factors that contribute to you doing your best, and you can objectively rate yourself. This will help you focus on the areas you want to develop. Factors could include:

- Mental preparation
- Nutrition
- Physical preparation
- Recovery
- Technical and tactical skills

The development of mental skills is just as important as physical skills but often gets neglected.

You can feel unconfident and perform – You can *feel* confident and not perform how you want, and vice versa. Shift your focus from feelings to your plan and process. You can still commit to your plan even if you are not feeling confident. Athletes that view pre-competition anxiety as understandable rather than debilitating are able to cope better. Lutalo Muhammad describes how you don't have to believe in yourself and feel confident all the time, "Just do the work and see what happens; it is okay if you are shy or have doubts. Learn to enjoy the training."

Communicate how you want others to support you on competition day – Those around you will be well-meaning but might not always say things that you find helpful. You can pre-empt this by discussing what you find helpful before competition day. You could tick the phrases below that you like, or come up with your own.

- Tell me how you are feeling
- It is understandable to feel like that
- Remember your strengths are…
- Let's go over your plan/process
- Focus on doing your best; that is all you can do
- Let's see this as a challenge and opportunity

Example competition day preparation checklist

1. Write down your ideal mindset
2. Face the fears and consequences you are worried about, finding answers that reassure you and allow you to adopt your mindset. Remind yourself it is your choice to compete
3. Write down your strengths, abilities, and preparation
4. Have a plan and focus points or words to help you stick to the plan
5. What does doing your best look like in areas such as physical, technical, tactical, nutrition, and mental? What is in your control that will help you do your best?

Frustrations

Sporting events can be a source of frustration; from refereeing decisions you don't agree with to delays in schedules. Being frustrated takes up mental energy and places more demands on your mind. Athletes often get frustrated by the same thing at every competition. Writing down what you find frustrating and accepting that these will happen will help you to choose a different response. The quicker you can let them go and *refocus your attention on your plan*, the better you will perform.

Dealing with disappointment

This is a great skill to develop to help you in life and sport. Disappointments are inevitable and happen when your hopes and expectations are not realised. If you challenge yourself, it is inevitable that you will experience failures along the way.

Acknowledge how you feel and name it – Be aware of the language you use. Saying you are devastated will produce stronger emotions than saying you are disappointed. Accept it is okay to feel disappointed; it means you care about what you are doing. As with all feelings, it will pass and fade away. You might want to give yourself a timeframe of when you want to move on. Talk to others and get support.

Realistic expectations – Following a disappointment, you can reflect on your expectations and where you set the bar. Aiming for perfection often results in disappointment. If you cannot do something in training, you shouldn't expect to do it in a competition.

Lessons – A helpful way to deal with disappointment is to objectively review what went well and what could be improved. Immediately after the event, emotions can cloud objectivity so wait until you can think clearly. When you feel disappointment, do you look inward or outward for explanations? Inward means you look at what you could have done better under the circumstances, whilst outward means factors in the environment. We want to avoid blaming and excuses as they don't help preparation for the next competition.

The journey is not linear – The road to improvement does not follow a straight upward trajectory. Sometimes, you will make big leaps, and at other times, you will plateau. Jonathan Wray has won the Superbike World Championship six times and has talked about how he *learnt to lose* as well as win.

As you move up the performance pathway, the margins between winning and losing decrease, so a small difference in your performance will have a big difference in the result. Learning to deal with loss is a key part of developing as an athlete. The *meaning* you give a loss is important; if you see it as inevitable and part of the learning process, you will be able to move on quicker. Learn to enjoy the process of improving, not just the outcome.

Perspective – This is an important skill for managing many difficulties in life. Remind yourself that sporting performance is not life and death. Having other things in your life that matter will help you gain an alternative point of view and allow you to focus on your plan for improvement. Hope is a feeling that can help you move forwards and focus on the future.

Lutalo Muhammad's story brings these aspects to life. It was the last second of the Olympic final in Rio 2016, and he was in the lead. Watching from the stands, it seemed like it was all over. His opponent Cheik Cisse had other ideas and scored a head kick before the round ended. Lutalo's gold medal dream was gone. "I was in the shape of my life and lost in the final second. As painful as it was at the time, the sun still rose the next day, life went on. Perspective and my faith in God helped me.

"Cisse is from the Ivory Coast and was the first gold medallist they had ever had. He has inspired a whole continent; I am not sure me winning gold would have achieved that, so I am happy for him.

"Over time, I was able to create a new meaning from the experience, and it is still a great achievement. I got a lot of emotion out in the post-match interview, which helped. If you don't want to tell someone how you feel, you can always record it on your phone or write it down to get it off your chest. I knew my family would still love me no matter what happened."

Personal life

When aspects of your personal life are difficult, they are likely to impact on your sporting performance. Athletes are not robots who can switch on and off at will.

Louise played tennis from a young age and found that when she wasn't happy off court, she couldn't play well on court, but coaches didn't ask about this aspect of her life.

Sometimes, sport can be a welcome distraction from difficulties in life, but often they can make it hard to focus and can impact on sleep and rest. It is important that demands from your personal life are considered when planning training and recovery. There can be a perception that coaches and other support services just want to talk about sport. A good support team will want to understand you as a whole person. Building trust and putting effort into these relationships makes it easier to share personal struggles.

Transitions

Transitions happen when things change in our lives. Changes occur all the time and vary in the impact they have on us. "There is nothing permanent except change."[54]

The ability to deal with change plays a big role in our mental health, and many of us find this hard – especially when it is not of our own choosing. It can involve losing something, which feels painful as we have a bias that registers losses more than gains.

Changes might include moving team, club, or coach, growing from adolescence to adulthood, moving from junior to senior/professional, through to exiting your sport. For those who develop a life-changing injury or illness, the transition and adjustment to a new way of living can be difficult and painful and involve grief (the section on loss in Chapter 4 discusses grief in more detail).

Resisting change is like swimming against the tide; you either fight it or go with it. To effectively embrace change, we need to recognise how we feel about it and acknowledge and work through what we have lost. Then, we can shift our focus to what we might gain from the change and the resources we possess to cope with it. This can be a slow process. Embracing change can involve managing fear and anxiety about the future, so the tools we have discussed in the sections above will help.

---

[54] Heraclitus, Greek philosopher.

Transitioning out of your sport is a change most people find challenging. There are three ways this can happen:
1. You decide that you want to stop
2. Someone else makes the decision for you (by not selecting you, releasing you from a programme, or declassification in Paralympic sport)
3. An injury or illness forces you to stop

Even if you make the decision yourself, a sudden change to a new way of life can be difficult. If you decide to stop when you didn't achieve what you wanted to, that can be hard to accept, especially if your identity is based on your sporting results. In research, the more dissatisfied rugby players were with their career, the more they suffered from distress and sleep disturbances after retirement. Whether sport is your full-time job – or not – you are likely to dedicate lots of time and energy to it, so you will feel the loss.

Even though you know, rationally, that there will be changes as you go through your sporting life, it can be hard to prepare for them before they happen. Athletes want to focus on being the best they can be in their sport. The badminton player Gail Emms has said, "I had the CV of an 18-year-old when I stopped playing at 31. You must learn how to apply the skills you got in sport to a different world. I wish I had completed more courses while I was competing, but I wanted to focus on sport and nothing else."

Sporting organisations can sell a dream rather than sharing the chances of success at the highest level. Only 0.05% of football players who join an academy aged nine will have a career in football. Of the 1.5 million youth players currently playing in England, only 180 will develop and play in the Premier League (0.012%).

Wayne Richardson is a trainer and mentor with professional and aspiring athletes. He says, "Some clubs are better than others at managing this process; I know of players who were told they were being released by text message."

Being released from a programme and having dreams shattered can be difficult to manage and, sadly, several young players have taken their own lives after being released. This has led clubs such as Crystal Palace to offer aftercare programmes to help scholars cope more effectively. Palace now offer a three-year programme that helps youngsters find a new club, education course, or job.

A transition out of sport can lead to a loss of self-worth and confidence. You lose structure, goals, the rush of competing and the social elements. The runner Andy Turner said, "I was buzzing the first few months after retirement; I could do what I wanted. Gradually, the new world crept in as I left the bubble of sport and I lost who I was. I doubted myself, which I never did while competing. I was used to a structure, and now I had to find a new one. I got some qualifications while I was competing, which helped, but it still took me years to figure out what I wanted to do. That drive to train and push yourself doesn't just go away, so I took up bodybuilding then boxing. It has taken me ten years to be able to train to keep fit rather than to perform."

Gail Emms said, "You give your heart to sport; it is not just a job. When you stop, it feels like your heart has been ripped out. At first, you enjoy being able to go out and eat burgers for a bit, then you crash. I missed the adrenaline and didn't know how to replace it. I saw my rankings come down and realised in normal life there is no ranking to see how you are getting on."

The cyclist Chris Opie's journey ended before he was ready. "I was told by email that my team would either fold or we would take a 50% cut in salary. I couldn't afford to keep racing, so I had no choice but to stop.

"Suddenly, your goals are taken away, and I struggled with depression with no support from the team. I feel governing bodies should support athletes exiting their sports as you might only be on a team for 12 months. I used drinking to cope as I wasn't enjoying my new job.

"With support and encouragement from my family, I got counselling, which was brilliant, and I wish I had done it during my career. I don't think you can ever prepare for retirement as it's such a big adaptation; it is like coming out of the armed forces; life is so different. I think it is why so many athletes attempt a comeback.

"It is hard to find the same passion. Counselling has helped me appreciate the great times I had while I was competing, rather than wishing I still had it and trying to re-enact the buzz I got from racing in other ways."

Marc Woods is a former paralympic swimmer. He said he had tendencies to feel low and that sport acted as a protective factor for him. Once he retired and didn't have the purpose, endorphins, and rewards and adrenaline from training and competing; he struggled.

Ideally, clubs and governing bodies should provide support to prepare athletes for leaving their sport. Talking to athletes who have retired from your sport can help you prepare for transitions, and benefit from their experiences. It is possible to fully commit to your sport whilst developing other identities, interests, and qualifications. Accept there will come a point when change happens. You might not be able to avoid the feeling of loss, but you can feel more prepared to find the positives in the new situation.

The meaning we make of situations has a big influence on how we feel. You can examine your relationship with change and develop the ability to see the future as a challenge and opportunity. Chapter 3 will help you explore your identity and self-worth.

Summary

- Stress, fear, and anxiety are there to help us survive
- Stress is when there are demands that cause you to get ready for action. Stress in the right amount with the right recovery is good for us
- There are three strategies for managing stress – remove/reduce stress, reinterpret the source of stress, or recover from the demands
- You can reduce the number of demands placed on you or reinterpret things so they don't seem as difficult
- It is important to turn off the stress response and become calm and relaxed

- Fear is the perception of threat in the moment, or the memory of a past threat. The fear response is to keep us alive and safe
- Focusing on the rewards and reasons why you want to do something can help reduce fear. Using your faith or facts and reassurances from others can also help
- Don't avoid the situation; instead, gradually increase your exposure to the feared situation
- Anxiety is predicting or imagining a threat in the future
- We can learn strategies to manage fear and anxiety. The best way to do this in the moment is with a breathing technique called the 'physiological sigh' (two quick inhales through the nose and a longer, vigorous exhale; repeat several times)
- Competitive sport can place demands on athletes, such as dealing with injury and illness, lack of confidence, disappointment, and frustrations. Learning to manage these improves enjoyment and performance
- Change in sport and life is inevitable. Learning to accept and embrace change will help you deal with transitions such as exiting sport

Managing injuries
- Get social support and keep seeing your friends
- Reformulate your plan and accept where you are; don't rush or you won't progress
- Develop your skills through visualisation and watching videos
- Seek out successful comeback stories
- Find activities that match your values
- Develop optimism
- Focus on the process when you return

Chapter 6: Physical and Mental Rest and Recovery

- Why are physical and mental rest and recovery important for performance and mental health?
- What can make recovering hard?
- What can help recovery?

The importance of recovery for performance and mental health

Common sense tells us that recovering from physical activities is important for an athlete. Life and sport place emotional demands on us, so it is important to monitor and recover from both aspects.

If you don't recover properly – physically and mentally – this can lead to overtraining, RED-S (Relative Energy Deficiency in Sport), or burnout. Burnout is when you have physical and emotional exhaustion, feel unable to reach your goals, and lose interest in your sport, which can lead to stopping altogether. Overtraining results in decreased performance and reduced physiological responses such as lower immune function, disturbed sleep, and increased resting heart rate. Insufficient recovery can impact on your mood, emotion management, and ability to enjoy life. It can lead to plateauing or decreasing performances, which in turn causes emotional distress. An explanation of what happens when we train and recover is captured in the footnote below.[55]

---

[55] Our brain and bodies constantly work for homeostasis – the stability of various systems that work within it. Stress disrupts this and recovery is the process with which we return to homeostasis. These stressors can be mental, or physical, such as the stress of training. In the short term, recovery occurs via: the replenishing of fuel sources (nutrition), rehydration, reducing inflammation, repair of soft tissue, and downregulating mental stress. Over a longer timeframe, to improve an athlete's performance, we apply systemized stress via training, which increases fatigue levels. Once an optimum level of fatigue is reached, this stress is reduced or removed, to allow the athlete's body to

The three-system model

This model shows that we can spend time in three emotional states – drive, threat, or recovery.[56] The threat state is when we see things as hard to cope with or unsafe. The drive state is when we use energy to engage with the world and get things done. Recovery/soothing happens when we activate the calming system in our bodies. When we feel under threat, we might work harder or longer as a way of coping (drive system) without spending much time in the recovery system. This is not sustainable and can contribute to burnout. We need to tip the see-saw back from alert to calm on a regular basis.

Here is an example that shows how you might start down the path to overtraining or burnout. You want to perform well and get good results. You have a training plan you are happy with, but sometimes push harder or add in extra sessions to get more benefits. If you must miss sessions because you are ill, injured, or have a life commitment, you feel anxious that you won't have done enough, and that it will impact on your performance. You find it hard to stop thinking about training and whether you are good enough, which impacts on your sleep. You always feel tired but accept this is what happens when you train hard. You haven't seen the improvements in training you expected, which makes you think you need to work even harder. Other athletes post on social media about how much training they are doing, so you want to keep up with them. You avoid social events and stop seeing your friends as much as you normally do. You have become focused on what you are eating, and it takes up a lot of your thinking space, wondering if you have got it right. You have started to reduce what you eat to be lighter. It is hard to enjoy days when you are not training as you are thinking about the next session. You don't

---

compensate, and hopefully an improvement in fitness to occur. Without subsequent further training, this fitness will also be transient, with the body returning homeostasis in time. (Rhys Ingram, Senior Strength and Conditioning Coach with the English Institute of Sport.)

[56] Compassion focused therapy three-system model https://www.compassionatemind.co.uk/

always tell your coach if you are feeling tired or have a niggle as you don't want them to recommend resting.

> *Activity*
>
> Think about your past week. Now draw three circles – one each for threat, drive, and recovery. The bigger the circle, the more time you spent in that system. How big is your recovery circle compared to the other two? If it is small, see the section below for ideas to increase it. If the threat circle is big, go to chapter 5 for ways to help you manage this.
>
>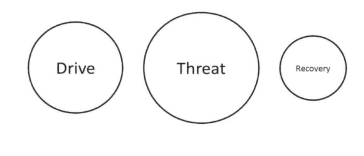

RED-S

RED-S is increasingly being recognised as a risk to an athlete's health and wellbeing. It is the result of not enough calories being taken in and/or excessive energy expenditure. It can impact men as well as women and can happen *without you realising it* by underestimating how much food you need, or the amount of training you are doing, or overestimating how much you are eating. You might be busy, so you are not getting the food you need at the right time after training.

The main sign is fatigue, and it impacts your hormones, immune function, bone, and cardiovascular health, as well as your mood. Athletes with RED-S often get osteoporosis which weakens bones, so they are more fragile and likely to break.

If you are not getting enough energy, you won't be able to sustain performance and health over long periods of time, are more likely to get injured, and have poor judgement and concentration. Male athletes can experience morning erectile dysfunction. Female athletes' periods may stop, which is a red flag that something is not right and could impact future fertility and health. It is not normal or acceptable not to have a period as an athlete. If you are on the contraceptive pill, this can mask this vital signal of health. Up to 80% of elite and pre-elite female athletes had at least one symptom, and over a third had two or three.[57]

Pippa, who we met in Chapter 2, only realised she had RED-S when she got a stress fracture. "I was experiencing tiredness and was given iron injections as no one realised what was going on. I thought I was eating ok as I was having three meals a day and snacks, and those around me had cut out carbs, so I thought this was normal.

"Coaches would talk about race weight, so I thought the lighter I was, the better I would run. I got glandular fever as my immune system was compromised. I had to stop running for a while to allow my body to recover and look at my relationship with food."

Pippa now supports others to prevent and recover from RED-S.[58] There is no validated screening tool for RED-S, but signs to look out for are tiredness, low mood, inability to train consistently, decreased performance, number of illnesses, relationship with food, and presence of periods (as touched upon above, if you are on the pill, you will miss out on this sign, so you need to pay extra attention to the other areas). You can be a healthy weight and still have RED-S.

Relationship with food

Your relationship with food will impact on your ability to perform and recover. This can exist along a spectrum ranging from:

- Normal/healthy

---

[57] Rogers, M. A. *et al*, (2021) Prevalence of impaired physiological function consistent with Relative Energy Deficiency in Sport (RED-S): an Australian elite and pre-elite cohort. *British Journal of Sports Medicine*.

[58] https://red-s.com/

- Athletic (the aim is to improve performance rather than having weight loss as a goal)
- Disordered
- Eating disorders

With an emphasis on weight and body shape, it is not surprising there is estimated to be a higher prevalence of disordered eating or eating disorders in athletes than non-athletes, especially those in endurance, weight category, and aesthetically-judged sports.

Depending on where someone is on the spectrum, there might be restrictions on food or certain food types, fear of gaining weight, bingeing and purging (being sick or using laxatives), seeing your body as an object, preoccupation with food, rigid eating patterns, not wanting to eat food you have not prepared yourself, body image dissatisfaction, and exercising to work off calories.[59] There might be a temporary improvement in performance if weight is lost, but it doesn't last.

You can have a body mass index in the normal range and still have an eating disorder. If areas in your life feel out of control, food can be an area where you can exert control. It can be a way of coping with past or present difficulties in life. An athlete told me, "Restricting food was my way of coping with anxiety; I was doing it as I hated myself at that time."

There can be multiple complex factors contributing to someone's relationship with food, so it is important to gain a complete picture. The mountain biker Evie Richards has spoken about eating disorders in sport. "I think it's hard when you're a rider trying to compete against people with an eating disorder as you look bigger, so that then puts pressure on you as you feel like you need to look like them. You must be quite a strong character to know that when you go to the start line, you'll probably be bigger than them, but you're healthy.

"I know I've struggled in the past, and I feel like it takes a lot of strong people around you to really encourage you that this is healthy; this is the way to be. I still think that in cross country, and

---

[59] https://www.beateatingdisorders.org.uk/

in all cycling and sport, that it's quite a common thing, really. When I first started, skin folds were so important, and power to weight was spoken about so much; but now, with my coaches, I haven't weighed myself in two years, and we don't even talk about my weight. It's irrelevant.

"If we do talk about fuelling, it's about, 'you need to make sure you eat on this ride', it's never 'right, you need to be a lower weight'.

"I really do think it's changing, but it's about more people talking about fuelling well, and how looking after yourself is important in having a long career."[60]

A positive coach relationship helps mitigate against things such as RED-S, and coaches need education and awareness to help discuss them in the best way. Pippa said, "Coaches have a huge responsibility and a lot of influence; we trust them. The things they say have a massive impact on our psyche. Comments such as you are looking lean can reinforce what you are doing, which might not be healthy such as cutting out carbs. You are looking strong could be interpreted as looking bulky."

Education and expert nutritional advice are vital to ensure eating is healthy and meets the energy demands of your sport.[61] There is increasing evidence of the link between gut health and how we feel mentally, which further endorses the importance of a balanced diet. Tests of bone and cardiac health can be carried out to check the impact on an athlete's body of their training and eating patterns. It can be hard to ask for help if you have a difficult relationship with food, but there is support that can help you manage this (sources of support are explored in Chapter 7). Restoring health should always come before performance and training!

---

[60] https://www.pinkbike.com/news/interview-evie-richards-reflects-on-her-rise-to-the-top-in-2021.html

[61] *More Fuel You, understanding your body and how to fuel your adventures.* Renee McGregor (2022)

Managing concussion

Brain injury through sport has received a lot more attention in recent years, highlighting the importance of proper recognition, treatment, and recovery.

Concussion is a type of traumatic brain injury that temporarily affects brain function because of a direct or indirect blow or jolt to the head, face, or elsewhere on the body. If concussion is not recognised or treated properly, or a second concussion is sustained shortly after the first, the risks of long-term consequences increase, and can be fatal.

A 5.8-fold increased risk of depression after 5-9 concussions has been found in retired male footballers. In turn, concussion can affect both sexes… recent research reported the risk of sport-related concussion in adolescent girls playing football was nearly twice as high as among adolescent boys.[62] Signs of concussion include:

- Loss of consciousness or deteriorating consciousness (you don't need to be 'knocked out' to get concussion as, in fact, the majority occur without loss of consciousness)
- Lying motionless
- Confusion, dazed
- Balance issues
- Changes in behaviour and emotions
- Severe or increasing headache
- Vomiting
- Double vision
- Seizure
- Weakness or tingling in arms or legs
- Severe neck pain (a medical professional should be involved in moving you if neck injury is suspected)

Sometimes, symptoms develop up to 48 hours after injury and can include sensitivity to light, visual problems, tiredness, or dizziness. Anyone with the symptoms above should be stopped from

---

[62] Levin, H. S. *et al*, (2021) Association of sex and age with mild traumatic brain injury related symptoms. *JAMA Network*.

carrying on immediately, and taken to hospital for assessment. They should not be left alone for the first 24 hours and should rest, avoiding too much mental/visual stimulation from phones/screens, and not drink any alcohol.

Katy Winton had a crash in 2018 during a mountain bike race, and the following March had another fall while racing in New Zealand. She told me about her experience of concussion. "My symptoms were more to do with balance than the cognitive side; I felt like I wanted to fall over when riding my bike. I had a lot of headaches, so I saw a doctor in NZ who works with rugby players and understands concussion.

"I knew I had to take it seriously as you can't function in life, let alone sport, without your brain working how you want it to. I wanted to get back to competing, but needed to be ok as a person first. I was told I couldn't push it, or I might not make it back.

"I forgot what normal life felt like; having headaches becomes the norm. It took a year before I felt like I was back riding how I wanted to. It was hard not being able to train, and I lost lots of fitness. I was nervous about hitting my head again after everything I had been through.

"My advice is to take any head injury seriously. Pay attention to what is normal for you in day-to-day life, so if you get a concussion you can pick up on subtle changes. I test my balance regularly so I can notice changes." Katy is racing again in the World Enduro Series, and they have produced a pocket guide to concussion for riders.

Recovery is individual, with most athletes recovering within 7-10 days, whilst up to 21% have symptoms after 30 days. It is an injury you cannot see, so it can be hard to accept and take the rest needed. Changes in mood, emotions, and behaviour are common, with many describing feeling depressed.

Sheela was knocked off her bike and is still getting symptoms 15 months later. She said understanding that recovery takes time – and this is normal – helped her make sense of what was happening, as well as talking to others who had been through the same injury. "Not being able to exercise (because it brought on headaches) was so hard as it is my outlet. Being given information about the physical, emotional, and cognitive symptoms helped, as I couldn't comprehend why I was struggling so much."

Melissa was a pilot, triathlete, and mountain biker. She had a mountain bike crash but didn't realise how bad the concussion was. "I've had to come to terms with a lot of limitations; I have to try and avoid brain fatigue, so I can't socialise or even talk on the phone very much, look at screens or bright lights for too long, or even drive very far.

"Even when I'm careful, I can still sometimes struggle to verbalise my thoughts or remember words. I've lost my career as a pilot and there's so much I can't do now, that I used to take for granted; it's been a massive change. I had to learn how to pace myself and give my brain frequent, proper rest time.

"It can be very isolating because you don't look sick, so getting help and support can be hard. At one point, I was depressed and had suicidal thoughts because I didn't know what was wrong and found it such a battle to get taken seriously. Learning about concussion helped me realise that I wasn't alone and that this was normal; it wasn't in my head (even though it physically was!).

"I learnt how important the mind-body connection is and started to be a lot kinder to myself. It's been a difficult journey, but I can honestly say that I'm happy now. You can't make changes and help yourself if you don't know what you're dealing with, so the more you can understand about concussion, the better."

Sport's governing bodies often have graduated return-to-play protocols that need to be followed once you are symptom-free. If you can complete each stage without symptoms, you can move to the next one. The first stage is always rest. For those with prolonged symptoms, social activity should be continued to help avoid feelings of depression and isolation.

The government's intention is to have a UK-wide rule for all contact sports, which would standardise procedures, to be published in 2022. Scotland already has guidelines for all sports, which offer advice for athletes of all levels.[63] Education is vital to

---

[63] https://sportscotland.org.uk/media/3382/concussionreport2018.pdf

ensure those around you recognise the signs and take them seriously.

What can make recovering hard?

Finding the balance between training and overtraining – Athletes and coaches are constantly walking the tightrope between the optimal amount of training and overtraining. This can be tricky due to the number of factors that need to be considered, such as life demands, travel, nutrition, the monotony of training, mental state, sleep, illness, etc.

More is better

This belief makes it hard to buy into easier sessions or recovery days. When you are active, you can feel more in control. It can be hard to equate doing nothing with making progress. Many athletes thrive on the feelings they get from exercise and can feel anxious if they can't train. The urge to train can feel hard to ignore.

Perfectionist beliefs

The belief that every session must be 'perfect', and missing or changing a session means your training isn't good enough, can increase the chances of overtraining.

Not being honest with yourself or others

This might not be something you are aware of, and it can be hard to be honest with yourself about how tired you feel or if you have a niggle. If you want to train and stick to your plan, it is tempting to ignore signs of excessive fatigue or low mood. You might not want to be honest with your coach if you think they will take you out of training or not select you.

Comparison to others

If you see other people training in a certain way, you might be influenced by them, especially if they are getting good results, even if this is not the best way for you to train.

Feeling you are letting people down

If you miss training or competitions as you need to recover, you might feel you are letting people down or not fulfilling your obligations.

Norms of the sport

Each sport has its own norms and customs. If everyone has always trained in a certain way, it can be hard to go down a different path. In some sports, traditions are passed down about weight and body shape that might not be healthy with the knowledge we have now. It might be culturally acceptable to be critical about body shape, and to encourage people to lose weight. This is a topic that needs to be handled sensitively and with expert knowledge.

Finding it hard being in the recovery system

If you are an active person, or someone who has a busy mind, it can feel uncomfortable or difficult to rest and recover. Humans tend to focus on what is most appealing in the present rather than thinking about future consequences. Deciding to go and train might make you feel better in the moment but not be helpful in the long term. Being on social media or watching TV can make it hard to go to sleep, even though it will help you recover. It can be tough to switch your mind off, especially if you have lots of life demands and difficulties to manage. Keeping busy can be a way of avoiding dealing with difficult thoughts and feelings.

Activity

Answer these questions to help gauge how you feel about rest and recovery. Are your answers and beliefs helpful in the long term? If not, what could you replace them with?

1. When I see a rest day in my plan, I feel/think…

2. The purpose of recovery days is…

3. On a scale of 1 to 10 (1 being hard and 10 being easy), how able are you to get into the recovery system?

What can help recovery?

- Mindset and beliefs
- Listening to your mind and body
- Post-competition decompression
- Sleep
- Flow activities
- Social connection
- Meditation and mindfulness
- Time in nature

Mindset and beliefs

Mindsets and beliefs are powerful. What we believe or expect will happen can influence what does happen. The placebo effect demonstrates this. A placebo is when you believe you are getting an active medicine but instead receive a sugar pill, and you gain benefits that you would expect with the active drug. This has been demonstrated with treatments for pain, depression, and cardiovascular disorders, amongst others. If genuine pain relief medication was given in a more hidden way (intravenously through a drip the person thought was saline), they reported less pain relief than a drug given with reassurances by a doctor.

This is fascinating, and scientists don't understand exactly how the placebo effect works, but it shows the power of beliefs on the body. In an intriguing study, individuals who thought they were drinking a high-calorie indulgent milkshake showed greater reduction in ghrelin (a hormone that makes us feel hungry) than those who thought the shake was low-calorie, even though everyone had the same milkshake![64]

In another study, hotel room workers were monitored to assess how much physical activity they did in and out of work. Those who were educated about how much exercise they were getting in their jobs – and how beneficial it was – showed significant reductions in weight, body mass index, and blood pressure

---

[64] Crum, A. J., Corbin, W. R., Brownell, K. D., & Salovey, P. (2011) Mind over milkshakes: Mindsets, not just nutrients, determine ghrelin response. *Health Psychology*.

compared to those who were told they were not getting much exercise.[65]

What the above shows is that the physiological reactions in your body are impacted by activity *plus* your belief about it. This doesn't mean that you can do a couple of minutes of exercise and get fitness benefits just by believing it is enough, but it does mean that your beliefs about your training will have an influence on its impact on your body. Knowing that beliefs are important means it is essential to examine those about your plan and training. If you believe you are *not* doing enough, and more is better, not only are you likely to feel worried, but it could affect the physiological impact on your body.

If you feel you are not training enough, or others are training more, get to the root of *why* that is. Is it because you don't buy into your training plan, you lack confidence, or you don't know how you will cope if you don't perform, and training is a way of feeling in control? Building a good relationship with your coach will help you have honest conversations about your training plan.

Once you have identified your fears and worries, address them with the techniques from Chapter 5. Examine your beliefs about the importance of recovery to check if they are accurate and helpful. Remind yourself that what feels good in the moment might not be helping you over the long term. If being busy or exercising is a coping strategy for difficult emotions, recognising this can be the first step. You can then explore alternative ways to manage your emotions, asking for support if you need it (see Chapter 7).

Learning to listen to your body and mind

This is an essential skill if you want to sustain health and wellbeing. It requires you to be honest with yourself and those around you. Are you able to tell how tired you are or which emotions you are feeling? What signs does your body give you that help you determine your energy levels and need to recover? Emotional difficulties will use up resources just as physical training does, so

---

[65] Crum, A. J. & Langer, E. J. (2007) Mind-set matters: exercise and the placebo effect. *Psychological Science*.

they need to be factored in when planning training. You might need to take *different kinds* of rest depending on the demands placed on you. Examples include:

- Physical – rest needed after physical exertion
- Mental – if you have been thinking or worrying about something, you might need to give yourself a break and find something to get engrossed in (see flow activities below)
- Sensory – getting away from light, noise, screens, or anything that puts a demand on your senses
- Social – taking a break from people who drain rather than give you energy and positivity

There will be times when training is supposed to feel intense, and you feel exhausted, but you shouldn't feel like that all the time. In Chapter 2, Katy Winton talked about her capacity to do things such as train, see friends, and smile. By taking note – each day – of her level of capacity, she adjusts what she does or tackles sources of stress.

You can start by making notes each day about how you feel, what you are thinking, and how much energy or capacity you have. Ratings of perceived exertion can be used to capture how hard you felt a session was, and the influence of your mindset on that rating (if you had a demanding day, you might find training harder, for example). You can think of it as a body budget, where you are making withdrawals and deposits and need to make sure you have enough budget left for future needs.[66]

For female athletes, you can learn how your period impacts on you – physically and mentally – and make adaptations. For some, it can be debilitating and have a big impact on levels of fatigue. In an ideal world, coaches should be comfortable talking about this, but you might need to bring up the topic. Pippa said, "When I am having a down day with my period, I know how to do damage limitation and not take it out on others. I see it coming and can put steps in place to help, such as having a bath or having an easier session."

---

[66] *Seven and a half lessons about the brain.* Lisa Feldmann Barrett (2020)

It is unlikely you can stick to any plan 100%; it is a starting point that needs to be adapted. There is no such thing as a perfect plan, so you need to challenge the perfectionist mindset. Accept where you are with your fitness and that plans will change. Be honest with yourself; are you someone who tends to do more, or train more intensely than the plan says, or are you someone who needs some cajoling to work hard?

Once you and your coach know your tendencies, you can acknowledge them when discussing your plan. Rhys Ingram is a strength and conditioning coach with elite athletes. He uses a poker analogy to describe the planning process. "A successful plan is a combination of skill (appropriately thought-out planning) and luck. At different stages of the game, we have information to make our bets. Based on the information we have, there is a higher or lower probability that our action is the right thing to do. Our cards don't give us the whole picture; nothing is certain. Just as the initial plan is based on an incomplete picture.

"In poker, you may call or raise in earlier rounds and then choose to check or fold as the cards are put down. In planning, you may need to change your plans as you see how you respond to changes in load or pick up niggles. There is variance and or luck involved in whether you win the hand (the decisions proved to be right) as the rest of the game plays out. All you can do is make the best decision possible, based on the information you have at the time."

It can be hard if you are not where you want to be physically; the key is to accept where you are and *do the best you can* with what you have. Trying to make up the training you have missed by doing extra is a recipe for disaster. Everyone is different and responds in a unique way, so focus on what works for you rather than comparing yourself to others. What people share on social media isn't always the full picture!

Those who understand sport know that plans change; you are not letting people down if you need to rest. Physiological markers can be used to help assess health and recovery and avoid overtraining. These include blood tests (measuring aspects such as cortisol, testosterone, and vitamin levels), heart rate, and bone density (dexa) scans.

Post-competition decompression

After a competition, especially one you see as important, taking time to debrief, work through how you feel, and make sense of what happened can help you recover. Having a process that you go through with those who support you after each event can make it easier to stick to.

Sleep

We all know how important sleep is for us to thrive. It is the foundation of good health and wellbeing. 'I will sleep when I am dead' might sound impressive, but those who live by this mantra pay the price. Overtraining often impacts your sleep, so it is a sign to watch out for.

Some people seem able to go to sleep instantly and rarely struggle, while others find it much harder, and it can be the source of distress. If you have difficulty falling asleep, waking up in the night, waking too early in the morning, or feel tired all day for several months at a time, speak to a sleep medicine doctor.[67]

Here are some strategies you can put in place if you want to improve your sleep. Experiment to see what works for you.

Routine – This is not always possible when travelling, but try to ensure you get up and go to bed at the same time every day. The temptation if you don't sleep well is to lie in at the weekends or hit snooze in the morning, which then makes it harder to get to sleep that night. If you do lie in, try to make it no more than an hour later than your usual time.

Light – The amount of melatonin in your system lets your brain know whether you should be asleep or awake. Melatonin is produced when there is darkness and is suppressed when there is light. Therefore, it is important to get daylight in your eyes within an hour of waking (ideally 30 minutes).

You could drink your morning coffee outside to help you get your light exposure. If you have travelled to a different time zone, getting outside in daylight in the morning will help you adjust. Reduce the amount of light in the evening when you want to feel

---

[67] *Why we sleep, the new science of sleep and dreams.* Matthew Walker (2017)

sleepy and have a dark room to sleep in. The light from a small bedside lamp can impact on the production of melatonin, with phones and screens influencing the quality of sleep we get. Some people wear yellow-tinted glasses in the evening to block the effects of light.

Adolescents have a different circadian rhythm, with their melatonin production shifting to later in the day, resulting in a reduced desire to sleep until late at night. A need for social connection through social media can also play a part. Later sleep means less desire to get up in the morning and reduced hours of sleep if they must get up for school or training. This reluctance to go to bed can be seen as deliberate rather than a function of the developing brain. Understanding this can help to work out a sleep solution that works best under the circumstances and avoid frustrations.

Environment – Create the best environment you can that is not too warm or cold; if it's noisy, wear earplugs. Keep clocks or phones out of sight/reach so you can't keep checking the time.

Naps – Only take naps if you can get the amount and quality of sleep you want at night, and don't nap after 2pm. Keep them short; less than 20 minutes is best.

Caffeine and alcohol – Consuming caffeine (tea, coffee, chocolate, gels, or energy drinks containing caffeine) after midday has been shown to impact on the quality of sleep. Even if you don't notice a difference in getting to sleep, it will still impact on the quality. Alcohol is a stimulant, and while it can help you feel relaxed, it is stopping you going into a deep sleep.

Timing of exercise and food – Avoid exercising or eating big meals too close to bed; ideally, have a two-hour gap.

Reduce excitement – You want to activate the calming system, so avoiding anything too mentally stimulating is best. Social media or screens often make it harder to relax. You want to associate lying in bed with sleep, so if you have tried to sleep for over 20 minutes, get up and go into another room until you feel sleepy again.

Manage worries – The more you can face and address fears and worries in the day, the less likely they will intrude while you are trying to sleep.

Breathing – Focusing on your breathing (for example, in through your nose for a count of 4, hold for 4, out for 4, hold for 4, and repeat) can help you fall asleep.

Plan what to think about in bed – If you don't give your mind something to focus on while lying in bed, it will give you something that might be unhelpful. You could picture your next holiday or imagine a relaxing walk you have been on. If your mind wanders, notice it and bring it back. Have a rule that you don't problem-solve in bed. If you need to remember to deal with something, have a notepad by your bed and jot it down.

Beliefs about sleep – Your beliefs about how much sleep you have – and how much it will impact you – are important. We are often not good at gauging how much sleep we have had, typically getting more than we think.

In research, people who believed they had poor sleep, and that it would have a big impact on their day, had worse cognitive functioning, reported more fatigue, and had higher blood pressure than those who believed the opposite. Many athletes do not sleep how they would like to before an important event, but are still able to perform despite this. The key message is to *do the right things* to give yourself the best chance of sleeping well, but don't let it be a cause of concern if you don't.

Flow activities

A flow activity is where you get engrossed in what you are doing. You can lose your sense of time, so you don't notice it has gone by. It should be an active rather than passive activity and not so easy that you get bored, but not so challenging you get disheartened.

Activities could include playing a game, painting, colouring, doing a puzzle, dancing, listening to music, or playing an instrument. Flow activities can help stop you from dwelling on something difficult that has happened in the day. Tom Daley famously knits during competitions to help him relax.

Social connection

Being around people who are calming, and whose company you enjoy, is important for recovery. Just being in the presence of others can reduce your heart rate and breathing rate. Not everyone likes hugging, but if you do, having physical touch from another person is a powerful way to connect.

During Covid 19 lockdowns, this was an aspect of life many of us missed the most. If you are not feeling good about yourself or your sporting achievements, you might avoid others, which further impacts on your ability to recover. Remind yourself that those who care about you are not judging you on your sporting achievements; they value you for who you are.

Meditation and mindfulness

Our minds often feel busy thinking about the past or the future and try to do lots of things at once. How often are you watching a film or talking to someone, and your mind has wandered elsewhere? Meditation is a practice where you use techniques – such as mindfulness or focusing the mind on a particular object, thought, or activity – to train attention and awareness, and achieve a mentally clear and emotionally calm state.

What is the difference between meditation and mindfulness? *Meditation* is the learning and training of the skill, doing it in a deliberate way, and setting time aside to do it. The more often you practise it, the better you get. An example would be practising focusing on your breath. When your mind wanders, you notice that, and bring your focus back as many times as you need to. This is called Focused Attention Meditation.

Mindfulness is putting this skill into practice in real-life situations. It is the awareness that arises through paying attention, on purpose, in the present moment, non-judgmentally. You are talking to a friend, and your mind wanders onto the next training session or the difficult conversation you need to have tomorrow. You can notice these thoughts and feelings, not judge them, and bring your focus and attention back to your conversation. It is harder to do in real life, which is why regular practice can help.

Most practices incorporate focusing on your breath. There are hundreds of different meditation and mindfulness techniques, so the trick is to find the one that works for you. There are apps available that can guide you as you practise this skill. You can then practise doing other activities mindfully, where you focus as fully as possible on what you are doing.

Mindful eating is a good example as we often eat without paying attention and don't really experience our food. Yoga and Pilates can also help you practise focusing on the present. Jade Jones said, "I do 10 minutes of mindfulness every day to practise being present, as well as writing down what I am grateful for. I find it has really helped me feel calmer."

Mindfulness has been found to facilitate general wellbeing and enhance elite performance. However, it is not for everyone; some can find it difficult or threatening to sit with their thoughts.[68]

Time in nature

There is increasing evidence that being outside in nature has health and wellbeing benefits, such as reducing heart rate and blood pressure and aiding sleep. To get benefits, spending two hours or more per week is the optimal amount of time,[69] but some is better than none. This could be in a park, by the sea, or anywhere where nature is present. The Japanese have a practice called *shinrin-yoku* (forest bathing), where they sit amongst trees while focusing on their breath. Some studies have found that blue space (areas next to water) offer the greatest benefits. If you take part in an indoor sport and your other life activities are also indoors, making time to spend in nature could be beneficial.

---

[68] Gardner, F. L. & Moore, Z. E. (2012) Mindfulness and acceptance models in sport psychology: a decade of basic and applied scientific advancements. *Canadian Psychology*.

[69] White, M. P. *et al.* (2019) Spending at least 120 minutes a week in nature is associated with good health and wellbeing. *Nature*.

Recovery area	Tick if this is an area to improve/focus on	Actions to develop this area
Helpful mindset and beliefs		
Able to listen to my mind and body		
Post-competition decompression		
Sleep		
Flow activities		
Social connection		
Meditation and mindfulness		
Time in nature		

Summary

- To maintain health, performance, and wellbeing, you need to prioritise the rest and recovery of your body and mind
- Failing to do this can lead to overtraining, RED-S (Relative Energy Deficiency in Sport), or burnout
- Worries about your performance, 'more is better', and perfectionist beliefs can lead to overtraining and poor recovery
- We tend to make decisions based on short-term rewards, and what feels good in the moment, rather than what is best for us in the long term. Awareness of this tendency helps us make better decisions for our future selves

- The following can help improve recovery – exploring your mindset and beliefs, listening to your mind and body, sleep, flow activities, social connection, meditation and mindfulness, and time in nature

Chapter 7: Support

- What are the barriers to getting support, and what helps overcome them?
- If you are struggling, what support is available?
- What can you expect from the different types of support?

What are the barriers to getting support, and what helps overcome them?

The understanding and acceptance of people struggling with poor mental health is improving, but it still doesn't always elicit the same attitudes as seen towards people with physical issues. A broken bone is simply not as complex to understand or help.

Attitudes can vary depending on your experiences, with depression and anxiety seen as more socially acceptable than sharing an episode of psychosis, for example. Due to the complexity and lack of definitive causes, there can be fear and discomfort when talking about or communicating with people with poor mental health. The response you get when you tell someone about your struggles will play a part in what you do next, and who else you might tell.

Not everyone will know what to say or respond in a way you feel is helpful, so it is important to try to find the most suitable person that you can. Athletes have been found to have more negative attitudes towards help-seeking than the general population. This could be due to the perceived costs of seeking help outweighing the benefits in traditional sporting cultures where you need to be seen to be tough.

Bradley Wiggins has spoken about this. "You're expected to be so mentally strong when you're an athlete. People say – 'oh you won the Tour de France; you must be so mentally strong' – but it doesn't correlate to normal life. I think a lot of elite athletes are insecure – I was very insecure off the bike."[70]

Some report feeling embarrassed about sharing their difficulties. On a rational level, we know all humans experience pain and suffering, but we can still feel alone and often feel that we should be able to solve things for ourselves. We might think that talking about matters won't change anything, or we don't know how to put how we feel into words or make sense of it. We can worry that we will get upset and feel out of control. It can be hard to find the energy to seek help if we are struggling or feel others are more deserving of help. We might not acknowledge to ourselves that anything is wrong, even when others check we are ok.

Cultural factors can also have an impact, where discussing emotions or mental health is not seen as acceptable. Fear of the consequences of seeking help – such as not being selected or having to miss training – can also play a part in the willingness to talk. Not knowing what help is out there, what it would look like, and the time and cost, can be barriers.

What encourages people to get help

If you have people around you who understand the complexities of mental health and openly talk about it, this can help, especially if they are open about their own emotions and struggles. This reinforces a sense of shared humanity, and acts as a reminder that we can all suffer and feel emotional pain. Hearing from other athletes helps to normalise experiences.

Lutalo Muhammad received death threats following his Olympic selection in 2012 and describes his experience of asking for support, "Stepping up and having a conversation shows strength, not weakness. I am a normal person, not a superhuman; if I push it down, it will come up even bigger at a time that is not helpful."

Being part of an environment that recognises the impact its culture and behaviours have on individuals' mental health is important. You don't want to feel like you are being sent away to sort things

---

[70] https://www.channelnewsasia.com/sport/cycling-dumoulin-courageous-focusing-mental-health-says-wiggins-2074736

out by yourself without those around you looking at the bigger picture and the role they play.

If you have relationships with people who listen and don't judge, you are more likely to talk about how you feel. It is good to know what the confidentiality boundaries are (who will they tell or not tell, and what they will do with what you tell them). Messaging someone to say you are struggling can be easier than saying it face to face. Being alongside them in a car or on a walk can also make it seem less daunting.

Athletes can be more likely to seek help if they can see the benefits of opening up, and understand how it will impact on training and performance. It is powerful to hear stories from athletes who have taken time away from sport to manage their difficulties and who successfully returned.

The cyclist Tom Dumoulin took a break from professional racing in January 2020. "I noticed that coming back from injury in 2019 was very demanding. Looking back now, for a couple of years, I was already on the edge of being physically and mentally done with performing every time and coping with my ambitions and the ambitions of the team and everybody around me. I think it was a weight on my shoulders for a couple of years.

"Last year, I'd struggled a lot already, and then in the winter I didn't recover any more from the season. I wanted to restart and build up for this season, but I noticed quite soon that I wasn't recovered, even after four weeks holiday."[71]

Tom took five months off the bike to recover and get support to work out who he was as a person away from bikes. He won a silver medal at the Tokyo Olympic Games and reports enjoying life and riding his bike again. This emphasises the importance of an environment that allows you time away from sport when needed.

Brief anti-stigma interventions and mental health literacy programmes have been shown to improve help-seeking *intentions* in elite athletes, although the *impact* of such programmes on help-

---

[71] https://www.channelnewsasia.com/sport/cycling-dumoulin-courageous-focusing-mental-health-says-wiggins-2074736

seeking behaviours is not known. It is argued that raising awareness is not helpful if the support is not there!

Ideally, sports/clubs should have information or provide support in the following areas:[72]

Prevention - providing education on aspects such as the mental health continuum (see chapter 1) and screening to see how people are feeling. Some athletes I spoke to said having education about how to understand and manage yourself, and your emotions in life – not just sport – is helpful. Many said it would be great if seeing a therapist was seen in the same way as going to a physiotherapist or strength coach.

Early identification – spotting signs that someone might be struggling, such as changes in behaviour, sleep, appearance, mood, or drinking excessively.

Early intervention – helping people early on in their struggles, or when they have experienced tough life events or injuries.

Specialist mental health care – being able to refer or signpost to specialist care when needed.

When to seek help

If you are experiencing patterns of behaviour, thoughts, feelings, and experiences that result in significant distress/suffering/pain/damage to health, or which are unusual and which impact on your life over a prolonged period, then support could be beneficial. There is no definite sign that you should seek support, so it is usually better to ask for help than not. Often, the current ways of coping are not working or are making things worse. What helps when you are feeling ok and want to maintain or improve mental health and wellbeing can be different to *what you need* if you are struggling.

Sometimes talking to friends, family, or coaches can help, but there may be times when you want more independent and professional support. Change can be hard as it represents the

---

[72] Purcell, R., Gwyther, K. & Rice, S.M. (2019) Mental health in elite athletes: increased awareness requires an early intervention framework to respond to athlete needs. *Sports Medicine*.

unknown, and it is common that part of you wants to address your difficulties, while another wants to avoid them or keep things as they are.

If you are struggling, what support is available and what can you expect?

Unfortunately, the availability and quality of support will vary depending on where you live. It is good to know if there are any support pathways that are available through your sport. Ideally, the support you receive should put you at the centre, and consider your past experiences, plus emotional, physical, social, spiritual, and environmental influences. Support should consider factors relevant to athletes such as overtraining, weight making, concussion and other medical factors that can present as mental health issues. Athletes' moods are influenced by how much training they do, so this needs to be taken into consideration.

General Practitioners (GP) – GPs can offer advice, referrals and/or psychiatric drugs. In England, referrals are often to the IAPT service. IAPT stands for Improving Access to Psychological Therapies and is designed for people with a diagnosis of anxiety and depression. You are likely to see a psychological wellbeing practitioner who follows a structured, manualised approach for 6 - 12 sessions. This will be Cognitive Behavioural Therapy (see below) or counselling. You can self-refer to this service without seeing your GP. You might also be directed to self-help materials or online courses.

If you are under 18 years old (in some areas, 16 years old), you might be referred to Child and Adolescent Mental Health Services (CAMHS), which has teams around the UK. There are doctors who specialise in sports medicine.

Clinical psychologists – Clinical psychologists aim to reduce psychological distress and enhance the promotion of wellbeing. They can work with a wide range of mental and physical health problems, including addiction, anxiety, depression, learning difficulties and relationship issues. As with all psychologists, they undertake a degree in psychology approved by the British Psychological Society before specialising in clinical psychology, completing a doctoral-level programme. They cannot prescribe psychiatric drugs. They might use a variety of therapies in their work.

Psychiatrists – A psychiatrist is a medically qualified practitioner who will have worked as a doctor in general medicine and surgery for at least a year. They will then have had at least six years of further training in helping people with psychological problems. They can assess if there is an underlying medical condition that might be presenting as emotional distress. They can prescribe psychiatric drugs, and in many cases, you will be given a diagnosis and be offered a prescription. They can refer you to others for psychotherapy or carry it out themselves. There are an increasing number of psychiatrists who specialise in sport.

Counsellors and psychotherapists – There is overlap in what both offer; for example, providing a safe, confidential, and non-judgemental space for you to talk about your issues and concerns, working on the basis that emotional difficulties can be helped by talking and that people can – and do – change. Some argue that psychotherapists work with people over longer periods of time, but that is not always the case. Counsellors can also be referred to as therapists. Neither can prescribe psychiatric drugs.

Counsellors work with people experiencing a wide range of mental difficulties to help bring about change and enhance wellbeing. The focus is to help you look at options and see things in a different way, helping you to find your own solutions.

Psychotherapists – Psychotherapy covers many types of therapy (see below), so the experience with a psychotherapist can vary depending on the approach they take.

To check the credentials of someone you are thinking of working with, you can look on the Professional Standards Authority website. It will let you search by the practitioner's name to check they are registered and accredited by the following – British Association for Counselling and Psychotherapy (BACP), the United Kingdom Council for Psychotherapy (UKCP), the Health and Care Professions Council (HCPC), or the Royal College of Psychiatrists.

Free services and charities – There are several charities that provide information and support, often specialising in issues such as eating disorders[73] or hearing voices[74]. Some charities, such as MIND offer local support that varies depending on your location. Each Local Minds service is unique and offers assistance, including talking therapies, peer support, advocacy, crisis care, employment, and housing support.[75] You can also access free or reduced fee psychotherapy if you are on benefits or low income in some areas.[76]

Types of therapy

Therapy is different to a supportive chat or a sympathetic ear. Therapy generally has a focus – mutually agreed upon goals, interventions to reach those goals, and ways to tell when they have been reached. During therapy, you should learn something about yourself. Occasional or unfocused conversations are not enough for changes and shifts to occur.[77]

For each type of therapy, there are studies that demonstrate a range of effectiveness. There are pros and cons to each type as well, so understanding what each one offers can help you make a more informed choice, and decide if therapy is right for you.

Therapists that draw on several different approaches might call themselves 'integrative' or 'blended'. Therapy can take place one-to-one (online or face-to-face), in a group, with your partner, or with your family. Group therapy can help you connect with others experiencing the same or similar issues, helping you feel less alone and more understood.

Some of these therapies will only be available in some areas or by paying to see a private therapist. If you feel accepted, understood, and liked by the therapist early in the relationship, it is more likely to be successful. You might not find the right person or therapy straight away, so it is worth persevering.

---

[73] https://www.beateatingdisorders.org.uk/

[74] The hearing voices network https://www.hearing-voices.org

[75] https://www.mind.org.uk/information-support/local-minds/

[76] https://freepsychotherapynetwork.com/

[77] *Beginnings, the art and science of planning psychotherapy*. Mary Jo Peebles-Kleiger (2002)

Below are examples of approaches you are most likely to come across, but this is not an exhaustive list.

Cognitive Behavioural Therapy (CBT) – This is a commonly offered form of therapy. This approach states that psychological problems are based on unhelpful ways of thinking and/or learned patterns of behaviour. It is not events that directly cause emotions and behaviours; it is our beliefs about the events. It is argued we can develop irrational beliefs that can cause us distress and lead to unhelpful emotions and behaviours.

The aim of CBT is to develop more helpful patterns and ways of thinking. For example, you might catastrophise an event – say public speaking – and think it is the end of the world. In reality, the consequences are actually not that bad.

From a behavioural perspective, meanwhile, if you are afraid of speaking in public, you might gradually increase the number of people you speak in front of, starting with those you feel most relaxed with. You are focusing on carrying out the behaviours rather than focusing on how you feel.

With CBT, you are likely to get homework and worksheets to complete between sessions. If you avoid emotions, this approach might not be as helpful, as it can encourage rational thinking with less emphasis on exploring emotions.

CBT has evolved over the years, with new versions appearing. These include ACT, DBT, and CFT (see below).

Acceptance and Commitment Therapy (ACT) – People are helped to learn to stop avoiding, denying, and struggling with their inner emotions and, instead, accept that these deeper feelings are appropriate responses to certain situations and should not prevent them from moving forward in their lives.

With this understanding, people begin to accept their hardships and commit to making necessary changes in their behaviour, regardless of what is going on in their lives and how they feel about it.

The creator of ACT, Steven Hayes, says, "We as a culture seem to be dedicated to the idea that 'negative' human emotions need to be fixed, managed, or changed – not experienced as part of a whole life.

"We are treating our own lives as problems to be solved as if we can sort through our experiences for the ones we like and throw out the rest. Acceptance, mindfulness, and values are key psychological tools needed for that transformative shift."

Dialectical Behaviour Therapy (DBT) – Dialectical means trying to understand that two things that seem opposite can be true. One example might be accepting you are worthy as a person and still wanting to change your behaviour. It is designed for those who feel emotions intensely.

Compassion Focused Therapy (CFT) – This therapy is often used with those experiencing high levels of shame and self-criticism. The aim is to develop a more compassionate inner voice, with compassion being defined as a sensitivity to suffering in oneself and others, with a commitment to try to alleviate and prevent it.

CFT explores the interaction between three human affect regulation systems: threat protection, drive, and recovery/soothing (as discussed in chapter 6), with the aim of dealing with imbalances, such as spending a lot of time in the threat-protection system and little in the recovery one, which can lead to burn out.

Psychoanalytic Psychotherapy[78] – This type of therapy focuses on understanding your relationships to help you live in the present rather than reacting to past experiences.

Ways of being that helped us survive or deal with challenges might no longer serve us and can cause distress. We often repeat these patterns without being aware of them. The psychologist Jonathan Shedler says, "Therapy works on the premise that we do not fully know our own hearts and minds, and many important things take place outside awareness. It is not just that we do not fully know our own minds, but there are things we seem not to want to know. There are things that are threatening or dissonant or make us feel vulnerable in some way, so we tend to look away."

---

[78] Shedler, J. (2006) *That was then, this is now: Psychoanalytic psychotherapy for the rest of us.* Retrieved from http://jonathanshedler.com/writings/

The relationship between you and the therapist is examined, as patterns in other relationships will be played out in the therapy room. Therapy seeks to understand and rework problematic patterns. This type of therapy also looks at defences. A defence is a way of separating ourselves from unpleasant events, thoughts or actions. This might be by not noticing something or distracting ourselves. Examples include denial, where we refuse to face or accept reality, and displacement, where we direct strong emotions to something other than the cause of those feelings. You might be angry with your coach and then take it out on a family member or friend. Psychoanalytic therapy helps us recognise the connections that exist between thoughts, feelings, actions, and events. It recognises the complexity and individuality of each person, so doesn't follow a standardised approach.

Systems therapy – This type of therapy looks at relationships within a system, such as a family unit, and the impact these dynamics have on the individuals within it. It might look at how conflict is dealt with and how people communicate. In the sporting world, this could be the coach-athlete dynamic.

Creative therapies – These therapies encourage communication and expression through art and creativity, such as dancing or music, rather than talking, which can help people who find describing their feelings or struggles hard. You don't have to have experience in these areas.

Eye movement desensitisation and reprocessing (EMDR) – EMDR involves using side-to-side eye movements combined with talk therapy in a specific and structured format and is often used with people who have experienced traumatic events. It does not require talking in detail about the event.

Signs of progress in therapy

Below are some changes you might see if you are making progress in therapy:[79]

- Greater attachment security/sense of safety in relationships (see chapter 4 for more details on attachment in relationships)

---

[79] *Psychoanalytic diagnosis.* Nancy McWilliams (2011)

- Increased sense of personal agency
- More realistically grounded and reliable self-esteem
- Greater emotional resilience and capacity for managing emotions in a helpful way
- Greater ability to reflect and understand own and others' inner experience
- Increased comfort in functioning both independently and with others
- A more robust sense of vitality and aliveness
- Enhanced capacity for acceptance, forgiveness, and gratitude

Athletes who use therapy

Sarah Stevenson, who we met in Chapter 4, has found therapy helpful as she adjusted to life without her parents whilst retiring from sport. "When I am not feeling present and not feeling any emotions – like I am floating through life – I can notice this and reach out for support to help me face this.

"It is not always easy to recognise it yourself, but I have learnt ways to do this. Talking and learning how to make sense of what happened has been so helpful."

Rachelle, meanwhile, describes what she learned in therapy and how it has helped her. "If you don't deal with emotions, they don't go away. I tended to bottle things up and saw crying as a weakness. My therapist said if you open the gates now and deal with them as they come, it is done and doesn't prolong it (I would prolong things for weeks or months).

"It took me years before this really sank in, and I got it; it is now second nature. I don't put pressure on myself to be happy all the time; I let myself feel what I am going through but don't let my emotions control me. If I validate them, I find it easier to deal with them and come up with solutions."

Chris Opie said he didn't notice how much he was struggling; he knew something wasn't right but didn't know why. Those around him encouraged him to get help, so he found a counsellor close to home. "This is the best thing I have ever done. After nine months, I thought I was cured but realised it is good to keep it going. I now go once a month. It is a lot of me talking with the counsellor's input every so often. There isn't a lot of homework. I found it hard the day after as there is a lot going around your head, but it does get easier.

"I wish I had access to this during my career. I used to use drinking to cope, but this has helped me find more helpful ways."

Michael Phelps has said, "I struggled with anxiety and depression and questioned whether I wanted to be alive anymore… It was when I hit this low that I decided to reach out and ask for the help of a licensed therapist. This decision ultimately helped save my life."

Therapy might not always be right for everyone, but it is helpful when others share their experiences so we can gain some insight into what therapy is like.

Psychiatric drugs (medication)

17% of the adult population in England (7.3 million people) were prescribed anti-depressants in 2017-2018.[80]

Discussion about psychiatric medication is often an emotive topic, with research showing both benefits and concerns. You will find professionals on both sides of the fence, some stating we have over-medicalised distress and are over-prescribing anti-depressants, and others who state the opposite.[81]

There are people with lived experience who say taking medication has been lifesaving, while others say it has ruined their lives (and lots in between).[82] It is important to be able to make an informed decision to work out what is right for you. Gaining understanding *before* you are struggling can help you make these choices.

A lot of the understanding of how psychiatric drugs work is partial, or speculation, and effects seen in one person can differ

---

[80] Public health England research, 2017.

[81] https://www.bmj.com/bmj/section-pdf/187887?path=/bmj/346/7907/Head_to_Head.full.pdf

[82] Gibson, K., Cartwright, C., & Read, J. (2016) "In my life antidepressants have been…" A qualitative analysis of users' diverse experiences with antidepressants. *BMC Psychiatry*.

radically from those in another.[83] This is also true of non-psychiatric medications.

Most psychiatric medications are not cures in the sense of eliminating a cause or reversing a disease process. They have complex effects, which are described as therapeutic or adverse depending on the value judgement of the clinician or the patient.[84] Each person must assess if the effects of the medication – including side effects if there are any – are beneficial. There are some people who argue the effects of anti-depressants are no better than placebo[85], while others say there is evidence of their effectiveness [86]. Many agree there should be more research into the long-term consequences of psychiatric medication as well as the subjective experiences of taking them.

NICE guidelines say therapy should be regarded as the first approach for mild symptoms of depression. If medication is taken, therapy is often recommended in tandem. If there is a waiting time for therapy, offering medication can feel like something is being done to help straight away or to provide a stop-gap.

The NICE guidelines state the processes that should be followed if you are offered medication:[87]

- Explain the reasons for offering medication
- Discuss the benefits (covering what improvements the person would like to see in their life, and how the medication may help)

---

[83] Awais Aftab @Awaisaftab

[84] *The medical model in mental health.* Ahmed Samei Huda (2019).

[85] Kirsch, I., Deacon, B., Huedo-Medina, T., Scoboria, A., Moore, T., Johnson, B. (2008) Initial severity and antidepressant benefits: A meta-analysis of data submitted to the food and drug administration. *PLoS Med.*

[86] Cipriani, A. *et al*, (2018) Comparative efficacy and acceptability of 21 antidepressant drugs for the acute treatment of adults with major depressive disorder: a systematic review and network meta-analysis. *The Lancet.*

[87] NICE guidelines for managing depression, draft, November 2021.

- Discuss the harms (covering both the possible side effects and withdrawal effects, such as akathisia which is the inability to remain still, or impact on sexual functioning, and discuss any side effects they would particularly like to avoid; for example, weight gain, sedation)
- Discuss any concerns they have about taking or stopping the medication
- Make sure they have written information to take away and review that is appropriate for their needs
- Share how they may be affected when they first start taking medication, and what these effects might be (awareness of possible increased prevalence of suicidal thoughts, self-harm, and suicide in the early stages of anti-depressant medication). Explain that some medication may take a few weeks to see any benefits
- When their first review will be – this will usually be within 2 to 4 weeks to check their symptoms are improving and for side effects, or after 1 week if a new prescription for a person under 25 years old, or if there is a particular concern for risk of suicide
- The importance of following instructions on how to take anti-depressant medication (for example, time of day, interactions with other medicines and alcohol)
- Why regular monitoring is needed, and how often they will need to attend for review
- That they will need to taper (reduce slowly) the amount of medication when stopping (you should never suddenly stop taking medication)

For athletes, considerations also need to include the impact on performance and potential safety risks, as athletes usually train at a higher intensity than the general population.[88] With some medication, you can exercise to higher core body temperatures without noticing, which has safety issues. Stimulants and beta-blockers are prohibited in competition, with beta-blockers always

---

[88] *Mental health in elite athletes.* International Olympic Committee consensus statement, 2019.

prohibited for archery and shooting (stimulants prescribed would need a Therapeutic Use Exemption).

It is important that the professional understands the demands *you are under* as an athlete.

Mental health emergencies

This is when you need urgent help, and there is a risk to yourself and others. It could include feeling suicidal, self-harming, feeling very manic, or experiencing psychosis, such as hearing voices or hallucinating. Below are places you (or someone with you) can access.

Accident and Emergency department (999) – When you arrive, you will be assessed (triaged), so staff can work out the best plan. There can be long waiting times before you get seen. Some hospitals have mental health teams, or they can refer you to a crisis team. They will be able to keep you safe while you are there and might give you medication. Depending on their assessment, you might be admitted to hospital or released.

Emergency GP appointments – This option is ok if you, or those around you, think you are safe until your appointment. You can call your surgery or 111 (free NHS helpline). They can offer advice and medication or refer you to a crisis team.

Helplines – (See the end of the chapter for helpline numbers)

You will get access to trained people via phone, text message, or email. The NHS has an urgent mental health helpline for each area for those living in England.[89]

Crisis teams – A crisis team can include people such as psychiatrists, mental health nurses, and social workers. They can visit you at home or at a community centre. Support will vary depending on the team, but they often provide advice, medication, practical help, and someone to contact 24 hours a day. This can help to keep people out of hospital, and in their own homes.

You usually need to be referred to a crisis team. There are also crisis houses that offer an alternative to being in hospital and

---

[89] https://www.nhs.uk/service-search/mental-health/find-an-urgent-mental-health-helpline

provide short-term care and accommodation. The charity MIND campaigns to improve the care offered in crisis situations.

Open dialogue is an approach developed in Finland and is starting to be used in the UK and more widely. It is a model of mental health care that involves a family and social network approach where all treatment is carried out via whole system/network meetings with the person always present. The family and social network are seen as key to helping the person. It is often used to support those with psychosis, with the aim of reducing the use of long-term medication and hospitalisation.

Planning for a crisis – Mental health issues and emergencies can subside and reappear, so having a plan in advance can be helpful. You could write these down on a card and let family and friends know about it. This could include:

- The signs that show you are in crisis
- Who you want around you, and what you want them to do and say
- What external support you want
- Things that need to be taken care of; for example, pets or children
- What would happen if you are travelling overseas (particularly in a different time zone)

Sports organisations and clubs should have a mental health emergency action plan (MHEAP) which outlines the steps to be followed and who should be involved. It should include what constitutes an emergency and clear procedures. The IOC mental health in elite athlete's toolkit provides guidance on MHEAPs.

Following an emergency, there should be a graded return to sport – as with a return after concussion – with the athlete's health taking priority.

Suicidality

Sadly, a fifth of adults have had thoughts of taking their own life, and 1 in 15 adults have attempted to take their own life at some point.[90]

---

[90] NHS, 2016.

Of those aged 18-34, more than 1 in 10 have attempted suicide. In 2019, 75% of deaths recorded as suicide were male. Those living in the poorest and most socially deprived areas are 10 x more likely to attempt suicide.[91]

Often, thoughts or attempts are about wanting the pain to end, and not being able to see another way to escape it. The person feels stuck and powerless to make changes, or feels they have run out of resources to deal with life. There is a lack of hope about the future. This can be due to feelings such as worthlessness, shame, or loss. In turn, it may stem from external factors such as life circumstances, poverty, being unemployed or being lonely and isolated. Social perfectionism (what we believe others expect of us) has also been found to contribute.

People often feel like a burden and try to deal with things by themselves. They can think others would be better off without them.

Asking someone if they are suicidal does not increase the chances of them attempting it, and the question should be direct such as, 'Do you want to end your own life?'

Most suicidal people want the pain to stop rather than death. Being kept safe while you have this feeling can allow others to help you see hope in the future. The Silence of Suicide charity[92] has a helpline and online resources dedicated to those having thoughts of suicide. There is also an app called Stay Alive that contains information, a place to record your safety plan, customisable reasons for living, and a life box where you can store important photos.

Summary

- It can be hard to ask for support. Reasons include the feeling that you are expected to be 'tough', that you should be able to deal with things by yourself, cultural expectations, not seeing how talking could help, and not knowing what to say

---

[91] www.mind.org.uk

[92] https://sossilenceofsuicide.org/

- Environments that recognise the role those in power play in individuals' mental health, and provide relationships that listen without judgement, encourage help-seeking
- There are many types of professionals, support, and therapies available. Understanding what is available and what to expect can help you make the best choices

Helplines

The Samaritans – call 116 123 free 24 hours a day or email jo@samaritans.org

Shout – text 85258 for a confidential text service for those in crisis, free with most major mobile networks

Childline – available up to your 19th birthday. Call 0800 1111 free

Young Minds textline – text YM to 85258 for free, 24-hour text support for young people

Appendix: Visualisation

What is visualisation?

It is using your imagination to picture yourself doing or feeling something without actually doing it. It is a more structured type of daydreaming. We can imagine real situations and rehearse how we want to think and behave.

What are the benefits?

The same neurons in the brain become active when we imagine doing something as when we are actually doing it. When we can't physically train, or are injured, this can be a great way to keep the brain pathways active and improve them for when we return.

Studies have shown that visualisation can increase self-confidence, help maintain existing skills, and imagery focused on skill development has been found to be as effective as physical practice.

What types of imagery are there?

1. We can rehearse race plans, strategies, and routines
2. We can rehearse specific skills (to maintain or improve ones we have, or to develop new ones)
3. We can improve feelings of relaxation, calmness, and focus before we perform
4. We can imagine achieving a goal or winning (to help with motivation)

How do we do it?

Often people use a script – which they have written themselves – to help visualisation. This helps them create images and words that resonate with them. You can write out your script or do a voice recording of it. You can get someone else to read your script for you and record it if you prefer.

When recording your script, think about...

- The purpose. Which of the four goals above are you trying to achieve?
- Where and when will you read or listen to your script? Before training, relaxing on the sofa, lying down, etc
- Which senses can you use – sight, sound, touch, smell? The more you can use, the better
- Keep the script short; just a few minutes to start is good
- Once the script is written and recorded, practise it regularly

PETTLEP[93] is an acronym which stands for seven key elements to include during imagery, in order to create the best image possible.

- **Physical** – imagine relevant physical characteristics. For example, what you are wearing, and the equipment you are using
- **Environment** – imagine the environment where the performance takes place
- **Task** – try to imagine details relevant to the task (e.g., attentional demands) and imagine at the appropriate level of expertise for you (don't imagine doing something that is many levels above what you normally do)
- **Timing** – It is usually best to imagine in 'real time', but 'slow motion' imagery can be used to emphasise and perfect more difficult aspects of a skill
- **Learning** – the imagery should be continually adapted and reviewed over time to match changing task demands and your experience level. For example, as you progress and master a skill, you should adapt the imagery to reflect the improvement in performance
- **Emotion** – include the same images that would be felt in the physical situation. However, try to avoid unhelpful emotions (e.g., fear, panic). For example, you would

---

[93] Holmes and Collins model, 2001.

imagine competing with feelings of confidence/ calmness/ focus
- **Perspective** – the imagery perspective can be first-person (through your own eyes) or third-person (like watching yourself on video). However, one perspective may be better depending on the task characteristics. A first-person perspective (or internal visual imagery) may be more beneficial for tasks including open skills and with a focus on timing. On the other hand, a third-person perspective (or external visual imagery) is preferred for tasks where form and positioning is important

Example script (you can tailor this one or write a new one)

- Close your eyes and start preparing for your event
- Where is the competition?
- What is the venue like?
- What do you want to accomplish with this visualisation?

Take your mind to competition day. Begin your pre-race routine. Notice your surroundings – the sights, sounds, and people.

As you are visualising your surroundings, feel how you are in your own body and looking through your own eyes, listening through your own ears. Feel the fabric of your kit against your skin.

See yourself warming up and preparing to perform. Absorb the energy and excitement of competition.

Now turn your attention to the correct execution of the skills you want to use. Watch yourself for a few moments performing solidly. See yourself having a good strong start. Imagine following your plan and performing how you want to, being in flow.

Then give yourself some challenging scenarios. See yourself making a mistake or responding to something that goes wrong. Notice yourself getting quickly back to your plan and refocusing.

Trust yourself.

In this moment, you are in control of your body, state of mind, and performance. Feel a sense of confidence and control while executing skills and technique. You instinctively know what to do.

Visualise yourself going through a few more successful scenarios.

Open your eyes and bring your focus back to where you are.

Examples of how sportspeople use imagery

A number of athletes have talked about how imagery helps them to perform at their best, including Andy Murray, Jessica Ennis-Hill, and Jonny Wilkinson. Jonny would listen to a pre-recorded script prepared by himself and his coach before matches. It would last about 20 minutes and helped him prepare for different scenarios.

Jessica Ennis-Hill found visualising each stage of the Heptathlon event – before the day started – helped her to manage anxiety.

The swimmer Michael Phelps would visualise things going well and things going poorly. "When I would visualise, it would be what you want it to be, what you don't want it to be, what it could be. You are always ready for what comes your way."[94] [95]

---

[94] https://www.yourswimlog.com/michael-phelps-visualization/

Other books that might interest you

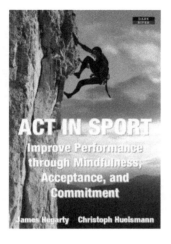

ACT IN SPORT: Improve Performance through Mindfulness, Acceptance, and Commitment

ACT – Acceptance and Commitment Training/Therapy – is a modern and effective psychological approach based on a scientific understanding of human thought and emotional processes. ACT uses a practical and easy-to-use framework for skill development through values-based action, commitment, defusion, mindfulness, and acceptance.

By utilising ACT, athletes will flourish into their better selves and improve their performances across their sports and beyond.

Tipping The Balance: The Mental Skills Handbook For Athletes

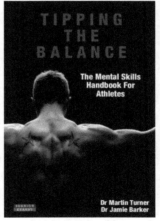

Tipping The Balance offers contemporary evidence-based and highly practical mental strategies that help an athlete to develop the crucial mental skills that enable them to thrive under pressure, perform consistently when it matters most, and enjoy the challenge of the big event.

This book is about empowering you – the athlete – no matter what level you perform at. In this book, you will discover the secrets of how the world's greatest athletes draw on cutting edge psychological skills to use what's between their ears to maximize performance.

Master Your Chronic Pain: A Practical Guide

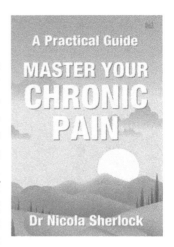

Do you want to manage your chronic pain and get your life back on track? Are you fed up with being held hostage by persistent pain and want to take action now? *Master Your Chronic Pain* adopts a holistic view of pain, looking at different aspects of pain management, from the benefits of mindfulness meditation to overcoming a fear of exercise to strategies for improving sleep. The emotional impact of pain is discussed, and practical tips for managing stress, worry, and low mood are given.

Togetherness: How to Build a Winning Team

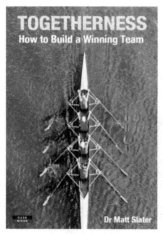

Togetherness is a powerful state of connection between individuals that can lead to amazing triumphs. In sport, teams win matches, but teams with togetherness win championships and make history. This concise and practical book – from Dr. Matt Slater, a world authority on togetherness – shows you how you can develop togetherness in your team. The journey starts with an understanding of what underpins togetherness and how it can drive high performance and well-being simultaneously. It then moves onto practical tips and activities based on the 3R model (Reflect, Represent, Realise) that you can learn and complete with your team to unlock their *togetherness*.

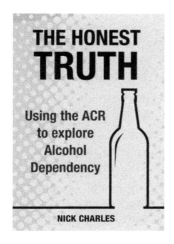

The Honest Truth: Using the ACR to explore Alcohol Dependency

Alcohol dependency – where alcohol has a hold over someone's behaviour – affects people from all walks of life. It can impact an individual's health, wealth, relationships, life fulfilment, and so much more. In *The Honest Truth*, we explore how to evaluate whether someone has a dependency on alcohol through the ACR: the Alcohol Consumption Regime. It is a focused, simple, six-week programme punctuated with periods of permitted drinking and periods of non-drinking.

The 15-Minute Rule for Forgiveness

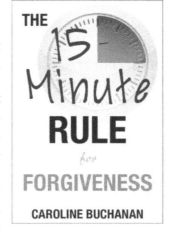

Forgiveness is one of the most powerful and liberating actions a person can take. Whether it is forgiving others, or yourself – for past deeds or mistakes – forgiveness can open people up to a life of happiness, fulfilment, and newfound accomplishment.

And yet, so many people struggle to generate forgiveness. Whether it is a partner who cheated, a friend who dishonoured themselves, or personal guilt that has haunted you for many years – forgiveness is hard! Yet, the power to forgive, and move on with your life, can bring untold rewards and enlightenment. *The 15-Minute Rule* is all about creating a safe framework for fostering forgiveness and self-forgiveness. We can all find 15 minutes in our busy lives and, through the short exercises and examples in the book, forgiveness and mental serenity can be attained.

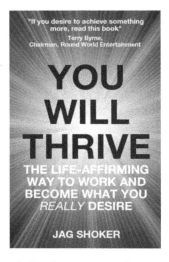

You Will Thrive: The Life-Affirming Way to Work and Become What You Really Desire

Have you lost your spark or the passion for what you do? Is your heart no longer in your work or (like so many people) are you simply disillusioned by the frantic race to get ahead in life? Your sense of unease may be getting harder to ignore, and comes from the growing urge to step off the treadmill and pursue a more thrilling *and* meaningful direction in life. *You Will Thrive* addresses the subject of modern disillusionment. It is essential reading for people looking to make the most of their talents and be something more in life. Something that matters. Something that makes a difference in the world.

All In Your Head: What Happens When Your Doctor Doesn't Believe You?

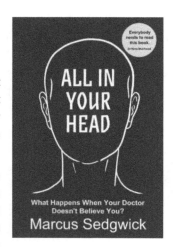

All In Your Head is about what happens when your doctor doesn't believe that you're ill. When they think you are imagining a serious ailment, or worse, faking it.

It's the story of the stigma that goes with invisible illness, and of the strange places that chronic illness takes you. It's the tale of bizarre treatments, and above all, the damage that's created through other peoples' doubts and indifference.

Lightning Source UK Ltd.
Milton Keynes UK
UKHW021408291022
411309UK00005B/79